Math for
Health Care
Professionals:
Quick Review

To my bride, Trisha. Thank you for being my best friend and partner.

To my three sons, Devin, Cody, and Lane. What a joy it is to see you three grow into young gentlemen.

To my parents, Kenneth and Mary Kennamer. Thank you for always being supportive in all I have done.

Math for
Health Care
Professionals:
Quick Review

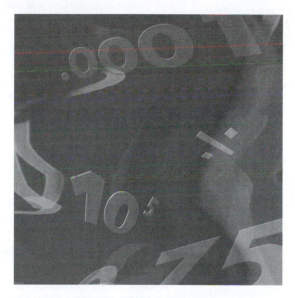

Mike Kennamer, EMT-P, MPA

Director of Adult Education and Skills Training Division
Northeast Alabama Community College
Rainsville, Alabama

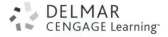

DELMAR
CENGAGE Learning™

Australia • Brazil • Japan • Korea • Mexico • Singapore • Spain • United Kingdom • United States

DELMAR
CENGAGE Learning™

Math for Health Care Professionals: Quick Review
Mike Kennamer

Vice President, Health Care Business Unit: William Brottmiller

Editorial Director: Cathy L. Esperti

Acquisitions Editor: Marah Bellegarde

Marketing Director: Jennifer McAvey

Marketing Channel Manager: Tamara Caruso

Senior Production Editor: James Zayicek

For product information and technology assistance, contact us at **Cengage Learning Customer & Sales Support, 1-800-354-9706**

For permission to use material from this text or product, submit all requests online at **www.cengage.com/permissions** Further permissions questions can be emailed to **permissionrequest@cengage.com**

Library of Congress Control Number: 2004049798

ISBN-13: 978-1-4018-8005-7

ISBN-10: 1-4018-8005-3

Delmar
Executive Woods
5 Maxwell Drive
Clifton Park, NY 12065
USA

Cengage Learning is a leading provider of customized learning solutions with office locations around the globe, including Singapore, the United Kingdom, Australia, Mexico, Brazil, and Japan. Locate your local office at **international.cengage.com/region**

Cengage Learning products are represented in Canada by Nelson Education, Ltd.

For your lifelong learning solutions, visit **delmar.cengage.com**
Visit our corporate website at **www.cengage.com**

Printed in Canada
5 6 7 11 10 09 08

CONTENTS

UNIT 1   BASIC PRINCIPLES

UNIT 2 ▶ APPLICATIONS

Chapter 8   Medication Dosage Calculations   /   153

Chapter 9   Weights and Measures   /   195

UNIT 3 ADDITIONAL LEARNING RESOURCES

PREFACE

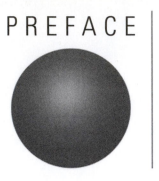

Math for Health Care Professionals: Quick Review provides a comprehensive, yet concise, mathematics text for individuals enrolled in, or interested in, any of the health care professions. It is written for those who need a refresher in math concepts. Written at a level appropriate for both secondary and postsecondary readers, *Math for Health Care Professionals: Quick Review* utilizes a unique competency-based approach in which individual abilities can be assessed and learning activities prescribed to support individual needs. Whether used in the classroom or for independent study, the organization and structure of this book meets the learning needs of everyone.

This book was written with both the instructor and student in mind. Instructors will enjoy the flexibility of selecting only the skills needed for each student from a cafeteria-style format.

Students will enjoy the easy-to-read format and will benefit from thorough explanations of each concept presented. Self-Assessment Post-Tests for each chapter, combined with Skill Sharpeners for each objective, offer practice opportunities for each skill.

ORGANIZATION

This text is organized in a logical fashion that moves from understanding the basic principles to mastering more complicated operations. These principles are then utilized to perform application-level functions that require both technical knowledge and critical thinking skills.

Unit 1 clearly explains the skills that are vitally important for health care professionals, and Unit 2 puts these skills into action with actual health care applications. Unit 3 provides readers with a collection of resources that will be helpful throughout their careers.

FEATURES

- **Learning objectives** for each chapter are clear and measurable.
- **Key terms** listed at the beginning of each chapter are shown as bold in the text and defined both in the chapter and in the glossary.
- **Skill Sharpener exercises** are offered after each section to provide additional practice on each skill.
- **Post-tests** offer readers the opportunity to assess their progress.
- **Answers** to the Skill Sharpener exercises and Self-Assessment Post-Tests appear at the back of the book.

ALSO AVAILABLE

For the Student

Math for Health Care Professionals

Order number 1-4018-5803-1

This book is intended for those without a strong background in basic mathematical principles. It offers more practice opportunities for the reader and includes chapters on how math is used in everyday life and whole numbers. Pretests are offered at the beginning of each chapter to help the student focus on potential problem areas. *Math in the Real World* illustrates the importance of mathematical skills to health care professionals.

Workbook to Accompany Math for Health Care Professionals

Order number 1-4018-9179-9

The workbook provides hundreds of questions for practice and mastery of each of the objectives included in the *Math for Health Care Professionals*. In addition, it can be used as a supplement to the *Quick Review*, as the principles between the two are similar.

For the Instructor

Instructor's Manual to Accompany Math for Health Care Professionals

Order number 1-4018-9113-6

This handy instructor resource includes answers to all the problems in the book, workbook, and quick review guide. It provides assessment and evaluation tools that will help instructors direct students to areas that require the most attention.

ABOUT THE AUTHOR

Mike Kennamer is a graduate of the paramedic program at Gadsden State Community College in Gadsden, Alabama. He holds a B.S. in public safety administration from Athens State University in Athens, Alabama and an M.P.A. from Jacksonville State University in Jacksonville, Alabama. He is currently enrolled in the doctoral program in higher education administration at the University of Alabama in Tuscaloosa.

Mr. Kennamer currently serves as director of the Adult Education and Skills Training Division at Northeast Alabama Community College in Rainsville, where he oversees a number of vocational programs including paramedic, pharmacy technician, medical assistant, nursing assistant, and home health aide. He is the author of *Basic Infection Control for Health Care Providers, Instructor Manual to Accompany Delmar Cengage Learning's Basic Core Skills for Nursing Assistants, Delmar's Basic Life Support Video Series,* and *Delmar's Advanced Life Support Video Series,* and served as scriptwriter for *Delmar Cengage Learning's Basic Core Skills for Nursing Assistants.*

ACKNOWLEDGMENTS

The author wishes to thank the following reviewers who provided valuable input on the content and structure of this book.

Linda Taylor, MT
MLT Instructor
Apollo College
Phoenix, AZ

Elizabeth McPeak, RN
Instructor
Southeast Regional
  Occupational Program and
  North Orange County
  Regional Occupational
  Program
Lakewood, CA

Donna Powers, RNC, BSN
Former Instructor
Health Occupations Education
Bound Brook, NJ

Cindy Pavel, MPA, BA, BS, MT, CMT
Department Coordinator
School of Health Professions
Davenport University
Granger, IN

Special thanks to the following companies for providing medication labels.

Eli Lilly & Company
Keflex

Endo Pharmaceuticals
Percocet

**Hoechst-Roussel
Pharmaceuticals**
Lasix

Luitpold Pharmaceuticals
Furosemide Injection

Merck & Company, Inc.
Comvax
M-M-R II
Mevacor
Singulair

Pharmacia Corporation
Celebrex

SmithKline Beecham
Infanrix

The author also wishes to recognize the valuable contributions of those individuals who participated the *Math in the Real World* features. Their experience and expertise is of tremendous value to the students who will learn from these professionals. Those who participated include:

**Laurie A. Romig, M.D.,
F.A.C.E.P.**
Medical Director
Pinellas County EMS
Pinellas County, Florida

Barbara Hammond
Radiology Assistant
St. Francis Medical Center
Grand Island, Nebraska

Mike Harper, CRNA, JD
Anesthetist
Gadsden Regional Medical
  Center
Gadsden, Alabama

Robert Lewis, RPh
Pharmacist
Bi-Lo Pharmacy
Trenton, Georgia

**Roger G. Wootten, AAS,
EMT-P**
EMS Instructional Coordinator
Northeast Alabama Community
  College
Rainsville, Alabama
  and
Paramedic
DeKalb Ambulance Service
Fort Payne, Alabama

As always, the Delmar Cengage Learning team was wonderful to work with. This project was signed by Acquisitions Editor Sherry Gomoll. Thanks Sherry, for always going the extra mile for your authors. Your hard work and commitment to producing the best possible product is much appreciated.

Initial work was handled through Sherry Gomoll and her Editorial Assistant, Jennifer Conklin. Thanks to Jennifer for fielding all my questions and for helping me to convert the *Math in the Real World* feature in the textbook from concept to reality.

When Sherry was promoted to Director of Career Education, this project was driven by the team of Marah Bellegarde, Acquisitions Editor, Erin Adams, Editorial Assistant; and Senior Production Editor, Jim Zayicek. Marah willingly listened to my input and concerns and kept an open mind when considering my suggestions. Erin was very helpful with early edits and formatting advice and did her best to keep me on track. Jim worked behind the scenes to make sure the project stayed on track and that each aspect of production went smoothly.

Thanks is also due to Judi Orozco of TDB Publishing Services, who provided the talent and skill that turned reams of computer-generated manuscript and my doodled notes into the attractive book you are now reading.

And of course, thanks are always due to my family, who continue to support and encourage me through the completion of each project I tackle. I could not ask for a better partner in this business, and in life, than my wife, Trisha. Our three sons, Devin, Cody, and Lane, are always a source of inspiration and often a much needed diversion from writing.

FEEDBACK

The author is interested in hearing from anyone who would like to offer suggestions or constructive criticism for future editions of this book. Contact the author through Delmar Learning or directly by email at kennamerm@nacc.edu.

TO THE READER

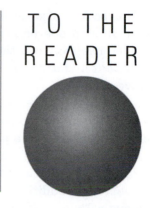

Welcome to the exciting and rewarding field of health care. Regardless of the health care profession you pursue, be assured that your chosen profession will be one that impacts the lives of other people on a daily basis. Your work as a health care professional will be valuable, and your studies in preparing for that career are equally important.

This book is a tool to help you assure success in your chosen field of study. The skills and abilities you learn through this book include some that you will continue to use in daily life. Please take the time necessary for study to ensure that you have mastered each of the objectives presented.

STUDY TIPS

You may find that this book is set up differently from others you may have used. Most books present a list of learning objectives and then cover each of the objectives somewhere within the chapter. This book is a little different in that it lists a learning objective, then immediately discusses that objective.

It is important to understand the value of objectives. Objectives are much like goals. In other words, each learning objective listed in this book is like a learning goal. Perhaps you can approach your study with that concept in mind. As you progress to each learning objective, make mastering the knowledge, skill, or ability in that objective your goal for that period in time. Work on that objective until you achieve mastery, then progress to the next objective.

This book is also set up in such a way that your instructor may tell you to skip one or more objectives. This may be because your instructor has evidence that you have already mastered a specific objective or set of objectives or because a specific objective or group of objectives do not relate to your field of study. Please understand that this represents sound educational theory but realize that you may, if necessary, work on objectives that are not assigned if you believe you need additional work in a particular area.

The accompanying workbook is very helpful in this regard and offers dozens of questions for you to practice. Please consider using this resource for additional practice that will lead to mastery of your mathematical skills. If you need a more comprehensive book, read *Math for Health Care Professionals*.

CALCULATORS

Calculators are a valuable tool and are used regularly in health care. However, a good health care professional should understand how to calculate any problem in this book without the aid of a calculator. If your instructor allows you to use a calculator, utilize it as a valuable tool, but also practice working some of the problems without a calculator so that you will understand how to solve problems when a calculator is not available.

Many of you will take certification and/or licensure exams as you progress in your health care career. Keep in mind that many of the certification and licensing agencies do not allow the use of a calculator during testing. Learn the requirements for the exam(s) that you will take and practice accordingly.

CONCLUSION

I hope that you find as much enjoyment during your career as a health care professional as I have had as a field paramedic and a paramedic instructor. Whatever you decide to do—whether you enter a career in health care or not—do what you enjoy.

Your patients will be able to tell if you really enjoy your work. Your attitude will reflect on the care you provide and how you interact with co-workers, your patients' families, and others you come in contact with. Let your patients know you care and that you are there to give them the best possible care.

UNIT

1

Basic Principles

This unit provides a stable foundation of mathematical skills upon which the student may build. Each chapter features a self-assessment pretest that can be used to better understand individual strengths and identify areas where further study and practice are needed.

A thorough understanding of the principles discussed in this unit will help in the successful application of these principles when presented in Unit 2 and in actual practice.

Numerical Systems

LEARNING **OBJECTIVES**

After completing this chapter, the reader will be able to:

- **1.1** List the common numerical systems in use today.

- **1.2** Convert Roman numerals to Hindu-Arabic numerals.

- **1.3** Convert Hindu-Arabic numerals to Roman numerals.

KEY **TERMS**

- Hindu-Arabic system
- numerical system
- Roman numerals

INTRODUCTION

Numerical systems, or organized systems for counting, are as old as civilization itself. For centuries, people have used numbers to trade with each other and to keep records. Whether they made scratch marks on a rock, or perhaps used pebbles or their fingers to count, people have used numbers throughout history.

Objective

1.1 List the common numerical systems in use today.

We commonly use the **Hindu-Arabic system** of numbers, though **Roman numerals** are still sometimes used. Although health care professionals are not frequently called upon to use Roman numerals, you should be able to convert from Roman to Hindu-Arabic numbers.

ROMAN NUMERALS

Almost 3,000 years ago, the people of ancient Rome developed a numerical system that is still used today, but only on a limited basis. This system has evolved from tick marks on a rock or the ground (as shown in Figure 1-1) into the additive system it is today. Numbers are read by adding and subtracting a series of symbols. The symbols used include the following:

I	= 1	C	= 100
V	= 5	D	= 500
X	= 10	M	= 1,000
L	= 50		

These symbols are combined to create any number. If a symbol for a lower number is placed before another symbol, the lower symbol is subtracted from the other. If the lower symbol follows the larger symbol, the symbols should be added. For example, by placing the I in front of the V, we subtract 1 from 5. By placing the I after the V, we must add 1 to the 5.

I is equal to 1	I
II is equal to 2	I + I
III is equal to 3	I + I + I
IV is equal to 4	V − I
V is equal to 5	V
VI is equal to 6	V + I
VII is equal to 7	V + I + I
VIII is equal to 8	V + I + I + I
IX is equal to 9	X − I
X is equal to 10	X

The same principles apply to larger numbers as illustrated in the following examples.

Example

$$X \ + \ X \ + \ V \ + \ I \ + \ I \ = \ XXVII$$
$$10 \ + \ 10 \ + \ 5 \ + \ 1 \ + \ 1 \ = \ 27$$

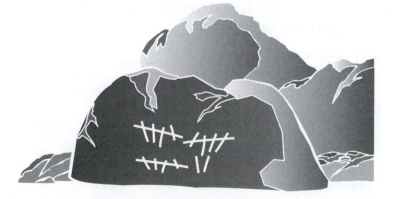

FIGURE 1-1 Roman numerals are believed to have evolved from something as simple as tick marks on a rock.

Example

MCMXXXIV

M	+	(M – C)	+	X	+	X	+	X	+	(V – I)
1000	+	(1000 – 100)	+	10	+	10	+	10	+	(5 – 1)
1000	+	900	+	10	+	10	+	10	+	4 = 1934

HINDU-ARABIC NUMBERS

The numerical system ordinarily used in the United States is called the *Hindu-Arabic system*. This system was developed around 600 A.D. in India by the Hindus and was brought to the Western world by the Arabs about one hundred years later. Today, we refer to this system as Hindu-Arabic or simply Arabic.

This system is based on the digits 0, 1, 2, 3, 4, 5, 6, 7, 8, and 9. By combining these digits, any number can be represented.

Objective

1.2 Convert Roman numerals to Hindu-Arabic numerals.

To convert Roman numerals to Hindu-Arabic numbers, convert the Roman symbols to Hindu-Arabic symbols and add or subtract as previously described. For example, to convert XVII to Hindu-Arabic numbers, first convert each of the Roman numerals to Hindu-Arabic as follows:

X	= 10
V	= 5
I	= 1
I	= 1

Then add these numbers to find the sum of 17.

10 + 5 + 1 + 1 = 17

◢ **SKILL** SHARPENER

Convert the following Roman numerals to Hindu-Arabic numerals.

1. XXVI

_____

2. DCLI

_____

3. DCI

_____

4. MCL

_____

5. CXXXVIII

_____

6. MCMLXV

_____

7. MM

_____

8. MMMDXL

_____

9. XXIV

_____

10. DCLX

_____

Objective

1.3 Convert Hindu-Arabic numerals to Roman numerals.

Convert Hindu-Arabic numerals to Roman numerals by using the same principles as converting Roman to Hindu-Arabic. For example, to convert the Hindu-Arabic number 129 to Roman numerals, first select the largest Roman numeral that equals a portion of this number.

C = 100

Subtract this number from the original number.

$$129 - 100 = 29$$

Now find the largest number that equals a portion of this number.

$$X = 10$$

Since X is the largest Roman numeral you can use, decide how many Xs are needed by dividing 10 into 29. The 10 will go into 29 twice; therefore, place two Xs to the right of the C.

$$CXX = 120$$

Subtract this number from the original number.

$$129 - 120 = 9$$

Since 9 can be represented as IX, add this to the right of the Roman numeral being created.

$$CXXIX = 129$$

SKILL SHARPENER

Convert the following Hindu-Arabic numerals to Roman numerals.

1. 145 _____

2. 3,420 _____

3. 312 _____

4. 453 _____

5. 1,394 _____

6. 1,250 _____

7. 38 _____

8. 365 _____

9. 3,217 _____

10. 333 _____

CONCLUSION

Roman numerals are not commonly used in today's health care system. However, it is important that health care professionals know how to convert between Roman and Hindu-Arabic systems if necessary. The remainder of this book will focus on the Hindu-Arabic system.

SELF-ASSESSMENT **POST-TEST**

Convert the following Roman numerals to Arabic.

1. IV   _____

2. XII   _____

3. MCLIV   _____

4. V   _____

5. VIII   _____

6. XXXVI   _____

7. XIX   _____

8. CXC   _____

9. MCMLXXXIII   _____

10. MCMLXV   _____

Convert the following Arabic numerals to Roman.

1. 2,003   _____

2. 14   _____

3. 98   _____

4. 3,456   _____

5. 231   _____

6. 798   _____

7. 465   _____

8. 2   _____

9. 72   _____

10. 112   _____

Measurement Systems

LEARNING **OBJECTIVES**

After completing this chapter, the reader will be able to:

2.1 List systems of measurement commonly utilized in the health care industry.

2.2 List and define key components of the apothecary system.

2.3 List and define key components of the household system.

2.4 List and define key components of the metric system.

KEY **TERMS**

- apothecary system
- English system
- household system
- metric system

INTRODUCTION

Health care providers utilize a variety of measurement systems, and combinations of those systems, in carrying out tasks such as medication administration, weighing and measuring patients, and measuring intake and output. As a health care provider, you will be called upon to use these measurement systems and to convert between systems.

Health care and medicine are as old as civilization itself. Ancient parchments tell of caring for the sick and injured. The measurement systems in use today include a combination of ancient systems, like the apothecary and household systems, and the more modern metric system. Tradition has played a part in the hodgepodge of systems utilized today.

This chapter discusses each of the three measurement systems in use today. While some are used far more than others, it is important to understand the relationships of measurements within each system and how each system relates to each of the others. Conversions between systems will be covered in Chapter 7.

Objective

2.1 List systems of measurement commonly utilized in the health care industry.

Three systems of measurement are commonly utilized in the health care industry. They include the:

- apothecary system.

- household system.

- metric system.

Though the **apothecary system** is not common today, it is still used in some situations and health care professionals should be equipped to convert between this and other systems. Measurements like dram, fluidram, and minim are examples of apothecary system measures.

It is important to be able to convert to the **household system** so that the health care professional can assist patients with converting from metric and apothecary systems to more familiar measures. The household system is also called the **English system** because it originated in England. Examples of household system measurements include teaspoon, tablespoon, cup, and glass.

Though the **metric system** is used on a limited basis in the United States, it is the system most used for medication administration. Milliliters, milligrams, grams, liters, and cubic centimeters are metric system measurements utilized in the health care profession. Each of these systems will be discussed further within this chapter.

Objective

2.2 List and define key components of the apothecary system.

The apothecary system is an old English system of weight in which whole numbers are represented by Roman numerals, and normal fractions are used to express fractional parts. One-half is sometimes expressed as "ss." This system is frequently utilized for measuring medication dosages using weight or volume.

APOTHECARY SYSTEM OF WEIGHT

The apothecary system of weight utilizes the terms and symbols illustrated in Figure 2-1. It is worth noting that in this system,

Term	Abbreviation or Symbol
dram	dr or ʒ
grain	gr
ounce	oz or ʒ
pound	lb

FIGURE 2-1 Apothecary units of weight

480 grains equals one ounce and 12 ounces equals one pound. In contrast, in the household system, 16 ounces equals one pound.

Therefore, you can expect to see medication orders using the apothecary system written as follows:

gr. vii	(7 grains)
℥ iii	(3 ounces)
ʒ ss	(1/2 dram)

SKILL SHARPENER

Write each of the following measurements using apothecary system symbols.

1. 3 grains

2. $\frac{2}{3}$ dram

3. 8 ounces

4. 4 pounds

5. $\frac{1}{200}$ of a grain

6. $\frac{1}{2}$ dram

7. 3 ounces

8. 2 pounds

9. 2 pounds and 11 ounces

10. $\frac{1}{2}$ grain

APOTHECARY SYSTEM OF VOLUME

The apothecary system of volume utilizes the terms illustrated in Figure 2-2. Though rarely used in today's health care professions, you should be able to convert between these and other systems.

Term	Abbreviation or Symbol
fluidounce	floz
fluidram	fldr or fl ʒ
gallon	gal
minim	m or ℳ
pint	pt
quart	qt

FIGURE 2-2 Apothecary units of liquid volume

SKILL SHARPENER

Write each of the following measurements using apothecary system symbols.

1. 4 minims _____

2. 1 fluidram _____

3. 3 fluidounces _____

4. $\frac{1}{2}$ pint _____

5. 2 quarts _____

6. 3 gallons _____

7. 2 minims _____

8. 8 fluidounces   _____

9. 5 fluidrams   _____

10. $2\frac{1}{2}$ gallons   _____

Objective

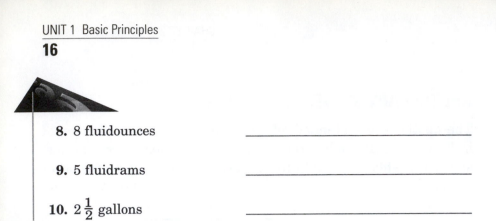

2.3 List and define key components of the household system.

The household system of measurement is primarily used when prescribing medication to be taken at home. Though the household system is not as accurate as other systems of measurement, health care providers must be familiar with it to instruct patients in taking correct dosages of their medications at home. Key components of the household system are listed in Figure 2-3.

Term	Abbreviation
drop	gtt
teaspoon	t or tsp
tablespoon	T or tbsp
teacup (6 oz)	tcp
cup or glass (8 oz)	C
pint	pt
quart	qt
gallon	gal
ounce	oz

FIGURE 2-3 Household units of measure

Objective

2.4 List and define key components of the metric system.

The metric system is used for many types of measurements in health care. Based on multiples of ten, metric measurements use whole numbers and decimals, rather than fractions, to express fractional parts.

METRIC PREFIXES AND SYMBOLS

The metric system uses prefixes that may be added to units of measure to alter their value. For instance, the prefix kilo-, meaning thousand, may be added to meter to signify one thousand meters. In similar fashion, the prefix milli-, meaning thousandth, may be added to meter to signify one thousandth of a meter. Other metric prefixes and their symbols are shown in Figure 2-4.

Unit	Value	Symbol
mega-	1,000,000	M
kilo-	1,000	k
hecto-	100	h
deka-	10	da
base	1	
deci-	0.1 or 1/10	d
centi-	0.01 or 1/100	c
milli-	0.001 or 1/1000	m
micro-	0.000001 or 1/1,000,000	μ or mc

FIGURE 2-4 Metric prefixes

Write the value that the following prefixes signify.

1. deci- _____

2. deka- _____

3. kilo- _____

4. micro- _____

5. milli- _____

6. hecto- _____

7. centi- _____

METRIC UNITS OF MEASURE

Metric measurements are utilized by health care providers to measure weight, length, and volume (Figure 2-5). Whether measuring great distances using kilometers or making miniscule measurements using micrometers, the base unit of measure is the same—the meter. Similarly, the liter is the base unit of measure for volume, and gram is the base unit of measurement for weight.

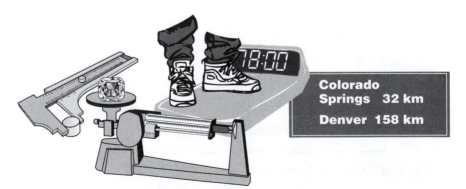

FIGURE 2-5 Though not widely embraced in the United States, the metric system is used for certain purposes, including health care and medicine.

SKILL SHARPENER

For each of the following, note whether the term is used to measure volume, weight, or length and whether the unit listed is a multiple of the base (ten, hundred, or thousand) or a fractional component (tenth, hundredth, thousandth, millionth) of the base.

	Measure of	**Multiple or Fractional**
1. millimeter	_____	_____
2. deciliter	_____	_____
3. hectometer	_____	_____
4. milliliter	_____	_____
5. milligram	_____	_____
6. dekaliter	_____	_____
7. microliter	_____	_____
8. hectogram	_____	_____
9. kilogram	_____	_____
10. centimeter	_____	_____

CONCLUSION

It is important for the health care provider to understand the relationships between each of the measurement systems. Though the apothecary system is rarely used today, it is sometimes seen. The ability to understand each system and its relationship to other systems, as well as how measurements within a single system relate, is important in the overall care of patients.

SELF-ASSESSMENT **POST-TEST**

Match the following units of measure with the appropriate system by placing A, B, or C in the blanks.

> **A** Apothecary system
>
> **B** Household system
>
> **C** Metric system

_____ **1.** minim

_____ **2.** gram

_____ **3.** tablespoon

_____ **4.** hectoliter

_____ **5.** fluidounce

_____ **6.** cup

_____ **7.** fluidram

_____ **8.** teaspoon

_____ **9.** grain

_____ **10.** pint

Decimals

C H A P T E R

3

LEARNING OBJECTIVES

After completing this chapter, the reader will be able to:

- **3.1** Define decimals.
- **3.2** Explain place value of decimals.
- **3.3** Explain advantages of using decimals.
- **3.4** Compare decimals.
- **3.5** Round decimals.
- **3.6** Add decimals.
- **3.7** Subtract decimals.
- **3.8** Multiply decimals.
- **3.9** Divide decimals.
- **3.10** Average decimals.

KEY TERM

- decimal

INTRODUCTION

Health care providers utilize decimals on a daily basis for anything from preparing medications to paying for lunch. Knowledge of the decimal system will help you to perform a variety of everyday tasks.

Objective

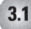 Define decimals.

A **decimal** represents a fraction of a whole number whose denominators are multiples of 10. For example, 0.65 represents 65 hundredths and could be represented as 65/100.

Objective

3.2 Explain place value of decimals.

Like whole numbers, decimals have place values. Since the digits to the left of the decimal are whole numbers, the place values are ones, tens, hundreds, thousands, and so on. The place values to the right of the decimal represent portions of one and include tenth, hundredth, thousandth, and so on as represented in Figure 3-1.

For example, the number 145.679 represents the whole number one hundred forty-five and 679 thousandths. One of the most common uses of decimals is in our monetary system where we deal with dollars and cents. Nine hundred sixty-three dollars and thirty-seven cents is represented as $963.37. Another way to say this amount is nine hundred sixty-three and thirty-seven hundredths. Using decimals makes it easier to recognize, add, subtract, multiply, and divide numbers with fractional amounts.

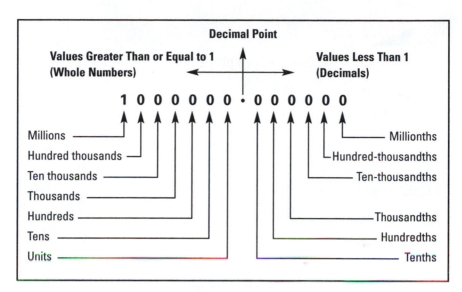

FIGURE 3-1 Comparing decimals

SKILL SHARPENER

Circle the digit in the one's place.

1. 123.00

2. 98.37

3. 21.938

4. 39.09

5. 2,222.222

Circle the digit in the tenth's place.

6. 56.9987

7. 884.09

8. 9,292.77382

9. 478,333.929

10. 993.909

Circle the digit in the hundredth's place

11. 8,437.0303

12. 12,267.009772

13. 487.0932

14. 9.341876

15. 4,576.888

Circle the digit in the thousandth's place

16. 637,367.8969

17. 988,989.434233

18. 895.2090

19. 57,847.0549

20. 20,009.00009

Objective

3.3 Explain advantages of using decimals.

Since the decimal system is divisible by ten, it allows for easy recognition, comparison, and calculation of very large numbers. Since our monetary system utilizes the decimal system, most of us are familiar with common mathematical applications used in making purchases, writing checks, paying bills, and balancing our checkbooks.

Write the following numbers using decimals. Then decide which is easier to read and understand: the way you wrote them or the way they are written here.

Decimals

1. One hundred seventy-five and ninety-eight hundredths

　　　_____

2. Seven thousand forty-three and seven hundred forty-two thousandths

　　　_____

3. Ninety-nine thousand three hundred forty-nine and sixty-seven hundredths

　　　_____

4. Thirty-three and ninety hundredths

　　　_____

5. Seventeen and seven thousand six hundred thirty-one ten-thousandths

　　　_____

Objective

 3.4　Compare decimals.

Decimals are compared by observing the digits in each place, beginning at the far left. Continue to the right until you find digits that are unequal. At that point, the larger digit represents the larger number.

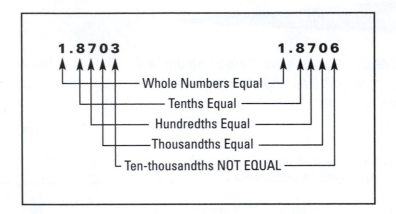

SKILL SHARPENER

Compare the following decimals by placing the greater than (>), less than (<), or equal to (=) sign in the blank.

1. 0000003.000003 _____ 0000003.0000003

2. 187.567 _____ 187.68

3. 65.76 _____ 64.78

4. 4,753.8473 _____ 4,753.74938

5. 7,483.1 _____ 7,483.99999

6. 9,485.09383 _____ 9,485.09384

7. 2,399.8940 _____ 2,399.894

8. 748.737 _____ 748.747

9. .5000000 _____ .5

10. 878.870 _____ 878.8700000

Objective

3.5 Round decimals.

Decimal numbers may be rounded in the same way that whole numbers are rounded. First, determine what place you will round to: the nearest tenth, hundredth, thousandth, or so on. Look one place to the right of the place being rounded. If this digit is 5–9, round the digit to its immediate left up one and drop all the digits to the right of the place you are rounding. If the digit is 0–4, leave the digit to its immediate left the same and drop all digits to the right of the place you are rounding.

Example: Round 345.9672 to the nearest hundredth.

The 6 is in the hundredth's place. Since there is a 7 to the right of the hundredth's place, round the hundredth's place up to 7 and drop all digits to the right of the hundredth's place. Your answer is 345.97.

Example: Round 45.27314 to the nearest thousandth.

If your answer is 45.273, you are correct. Since the digit to the right of the thousandth's place is less than 5, leave the thousandth's place the same and drop the digits to the right.

SKILL SHARPENER

Round to the nearest tenth.

1. 843.839 _____

2. 7,483.09 _____

3. 728.89 _____

4. 97.09 _____

5. 13.435 _____

Round to the nearest hundredth.

6. 8,437.48394 _____

7. 38,378.89384 _____

8. 22.2222 _____

9. 43.432 _____

10. 4,903.695 _____

Round to the nearest thousandth.

11. 78.93899 _____

12. 5,874.9806 _____

13. 93,939.065555 _____

14. 8,097.324132 _____

15. 8,439.5241 _____

Objective

3.6 Add decimals.

Decimals are added like whole numbers. To set up the problem, line up the decimals and add normally. Bring the decimal straight down.

The problem:

$$72.8 + 3.1 = \text{_____}$$

Set up as:

$$72.8$$
$$+\ 3.1$$

Add as you would whole numbers.

$$72.8$$
$$+\ 3.1$$
$$75.9$$

Solution: $72.8 + 3.1 = 75.9$

SKILL SHARPENER

Add the following decimals.

1. $4.5 + 8.4 =$ _____

2. $3.2 + 8.6 =$ _____

3. $89.22 + 77.56 =$ _____

4. $584.9 + 784.99 =$ _____

5. $232.64 + 346.98 =$ _____

6. 674.854
   $+\ 84.874$

7. 6.7
8.9
2.8
9.0
+ 4.5

8. 747.748
848.398
+ 8,327.82

9. 777.9
878.8
+ 7,832.378

10. 2.3
5.6
+ 7.9

Objective

3.7 Subtract decimals.

Set up the problem with decimals aligned. Subtract as you would a whole number, borrowing when necessary. Bring the decimal straight down to reveal the answer.

The problem:

$$48.2 - 7.1 = \underline{\hspace{2cm}}$$

Set up as:

48.2
−   7.1

Subtract as you would whole numbers.

48.2
−   7.1
41.1

Solution: 48.2 − 7.1 = 41.1

SKILL SHARPENER

Subtract the following decimals.

1. 5.6
   − 3.2

2. 8,774.885
   − 784.44

3. 8,889.33
   − 4,332.43

4. 14.5
   − 5.2

5. 100,982.292
   − 94,398.99

6. 889.94
   − 757.88

7. 5,894.94 − 4,783.84 = _____

8. 849.849 − 58.84 = _____

9. 954.9 − 944.98 = _____

10. 8,754.94 − 88.8 = _____

Objective

3.8 Multiply decimals.

Set up your problems as you would whole numbers. Decimals do not need to be aligned. Multiply normally. Count the combined number of decimal places in the factors and move the decimal in your product from right to left that number of places.

The problem:

$$12.8 \times 1.3 = \underline{\hspace{2cm}}$$

Set up as:

$$\begin{array}{r} 12.8 \\ \times \ \ 1.3 \\ \hline \end{array}$$

Multiply as you would whole numbers.

$$\begin{array}{r} 12.8 \\ \times \ \ 1.3 \\ \hline 384 \\ 128 \ \ \\ \hline 1664 \end{array}$$

Move decimal to the left the total number of places in the factors.

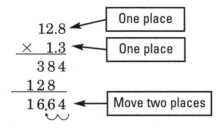

Solution: $12.8 \times 1.3 = 16.64$

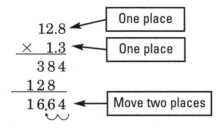

SKILL SHARPENER

Multiply the following decimals.

1. $89.54 \times 849.84 =$ _____

2. $8,493.4839 \times 884.489 =$ _____

3. $933.84 \times 944.3789 =$ _____

4. $448.84 \times 8,493.389 =$ _____

5. 9,389.84	**6.** 893.2283	**7.** 490.09
$\times$ 493.847	$\times$ 89.493	$\times$ 84.84

8. 3.4	**9.** 9,039.49	**10.** 895,849.9595
$\times$ 44.7	$\times$ 748.8	$\times$ 7,584.89389

Objective

3.9 Divide decimals.

To divide decimals, set up your problem as shown here.

The problem:

$$59.15 \div 6.5 = \underline{}$$

Set up equation as:

$$6.5 \overline{\smash{)}59.15}$$

Move decimal in the divisor to the right to make the divisor a whole number. Then move the decimal in the dividend to the right the same number of places.

Place decimal on answer line.

$$6.5 \overline{\smash{)}59.15}$$

Divide as you would whole numbers.

```
       9.1
  65 ) 591.5
       585
        65
        65
        00
```

Solution: $59.15 \div 6.5 = 9.1$

SKILL SHARPENER

Divide the following decimals.

  1. $8,877.9 \div 6.25 =$ _____

2. $4{,}355.5 \div 12.5 =$ _____

3. $15.35 \div 0.5 =$ _____

4. $848.59 \div 100.2 =$ _____

5. $12.1 \overline{)36.48}$ _____

6. $6.25 \overline{)98.1}$ _____

7. $8.94 \overline{)89.4}$ _____

8. $4 \overline{)38.65}$ _____

9. $5\,\overline{)\,485.625}$ _____

10. $3\,\overline{)\,90.54}$ _____

Objective

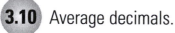 Average decimals.

To average decimals, first find the sum of the numbers in the set. Then, divide that sum by the quantity of numbers in the set. This is your average.

The problem:

Average the following set of numbers: 90.3, 92.1, 91.3, 94.8.

Set up equation as:

$$
\begin{array}{r}
90.3 \\
92.1 \\
91.3 \\
+\ 94.8 \\
\end{array}
$$

Find the sum.

$$
\begin{array}{r}
{\scriptstyle 1} \\
90.3 \\
92.1 \\
91.3 \\
+\ 94.8 \\
\hline
368.5 \\
\end{array}
$$

Divide the sum by the quantity of numbers in the set.

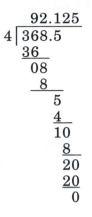

```
        92.125
    4 ) 368.5
        36
        08
         8
         5
         4
        10
         8
        20
        20
         0
```

Solution: 92.125

Average the following numbers.

1. 6.7, 6.8, 6.4, 5.9   _____

2. 344.4, 345.2, 341.5, 339.8   _____

3. 1.1, 2.7, 4.7, 8.5, 3.6   _____

4. 4,555.554, 4,557.552, 4,549.553   _____

5. 18.9, 20.3, 17.5, 21.7, 17.3   _____

6. 90.3, 100, 99.9, 94.4, 96.7, 98.3   _____

7. 55.5, 53.6, 52.9, 56.7   _____

8. 6.5, 10.8, 5.3, 7.9, 9.9 _____

9. 7.8, 9.0, 8.4, 5.3, 7.4 _____

10. 433.66, 434.5, 430.8, 436.8 _____

CONCLUSION

Decimals are part of everyday life. Whether you are paying bills, buying lunch, mixing or administering medications, or reviewing your paycheck for accuracy, you will utilize your knowledge of the decimal system. This knowledge and the skills you have learned in this chapter will help you to function better, not only in your job, but also in everyday life.

SELF-ASSESSMENT **POST-TEST**

Circle the digit found in the one's place.

1. 45.34

2. 690.00

3. 212.932

4. 32.893

5. 785.112

Circle the digit found in the tenth's place.

6. 54.980

7. 6,790.3532

8. 356.121

9. 100.56

10. 4,341.5550

Circle the digit found in the hundredth's place.

11. 34.1230

12. 500.3209

13. 65.9010

14. 750.8793

15. 3,500.5300

Circle the digit in the thousandth's place.

16. 540.3421

17. 442.3928

18. 7,988.8897

19. 452.5203

20. 32,321.902

Compare the following numbers by placing the greater than (>), less than (<), or equal to (=) sign in the blank.

21. 325.99 _____ 392.343

22. 25.11 _____ 25.1100

23. 65.120 _____ 65.12

24. 900.01 _____ 901.100

25. 645.321 _____ 645.0321

26. 7.9500 _____ 7.905

27. 81.245 _____ 81.0245

28. 9.012 _____ 9.0120

29. 34.321 _____ 34.3211

30. 90.09 _____ 90.090

Round the following numbers to the nearest tenth.

31. 34.3254 _____

32. 12.393 _____

33. 453.9044 _____

34. 45.433 _____

35. 475.755 _____

42

Round the following numbers to the nearest hundredth.

36. 8,347.474 _____

37. 34.32221 _____

38. 455.4454 _____

39. 499.9595 _____

40. 595.5943 _____

Round the following numbers to the nearest thousandth.

41. 3,433.33434 _____

42. 44.40404 _____

43. 434.4443 _____

44. 8.6452 _____

45. 0.3331 _____

Add the following.

46. 34.32 + 343.23 = _____

47. 454.32 + 32.01 = _____

48. 904.432 + 323.333 = _____

49. 9.343 + 45.433 = _____

50. 354,334.3984 + 12.3 = _____

Subtract the following.

51. 34.532   **52.** 5.440
  − 0.543   − 2.333

53.   975.431
        $-$ 543.94943

54. 90.43
       $-$ 89.49

55. 454.342
      $-$ 398.329

Multiply the following.

56. $747.12 \times 94 =$ _____

57. $9.03 \times 12.2 =$ _____

58. $453,439.9334 \times 393.49332 =$ _____

59. $4,543.3444 \times 93,030.9302 =$ _____

60. $373.39383 \times 990.3 =$ _____

Divide the following.

61. $3.22 \overline{)12}$ _____

62. $323.32 \overline{\smash{\big)}\ 493}$ _____

63. $89 \overline{\smash{\big)}\ 121.200}$ _____

64. $39.30 \overline{\smash{\big)}\ 334.332}$ _____

65. $32.1 \overline{\smash{\big)}\ 398.39}$ _____

Average the following sets of numbers.

66. 23.323, 34.3, 454.432, 984.422, 94.43   _____

67. 83.32, 304.03, 12.51, 34.343, 329.43   _____

68. 90.322, 91.323, 89.998, 93.23   _____

69. 765.42, 764.66, 464.44, 65.422   _____

70. 911.21, 900.21, 901.22, 890.322, 900.21   _____

Fractions

LEARNING **OBJECTIVES**

After completing this chapter, the reader will be able to:

- **4.1** Define fractions.
- **4.2** Explain advantages of using fractions.
- **4.3** Find the numerator.
- **4.4** Find the denominator.
- **4.5** Order fractions.
- **4.6** Add fractions with common denominators.
- **4.7** Subtract fractions with common denominators.
- **4.8** Define mixed number.
- **4.9** Add mixed numbers with common denominators.
- **4.10** Subtract mixed numbers with common denominators.

KEY **TERMS**

- canceling
- common denominator
- common factor
- denominator
- factor
- fraction
- greatest common factor (GCF)
- improper fraction
- least common denominator (LCD)
- least common multiple (LCM)
- mixed number
- multiple
- numerator
- proper fraction
- uncommon denominator
- uncommon factor

LEARNING **OBJECTIVES** (continued)

4.11 Define factors.

4.12 Find common factors.

4.13 Find the greatest common factor.

4.14 Reduce fractions.

4.15 Define proper fraction.

4.16 Define improper fraction.

4.17 Change improper fractions to proper fractions.

4.18 Define multiple.

4.19 Define least common multiple.

4.20 Find the least common denominator.

4.21 Add fractions with uncommon denominators.

4.22 Subtract fractions with uncommon denominators.

4.23 Use borrowing to subtract fractions.

4.24 Change mixed numbers to improper fractions.

4.25 Multiply fractions.

4.26 Multiply fractions using canceling.

4.27 Multiply fractions and whole numbers.

4.28 Multiply fractions and mixed numbers.

4.29 Divide fractions.

INTRODUCTION

As a health care provider, you may see and use fractions on a daily basis. Whether you are preparing medication dosages for patients in an emergency department or measuring height and weight of residents in an extended care facility, the ability to understand fractions will help make your job easier.

Objective

 Define fractions.

A **fraction** represents a part of a whole. For example, one-half of a pie is shown as $\frac{1}{2}$ and one-eighth of a pizza is shown as $\frac{1}{8}$. Fractions also provide a way to divide items as shown in the following example.

Example

> Five friends decide to split a pizza. If the pizza is divided into 10 equal slices, each of the 5 friends will get an equal share of two slices, as illustrated in Figure 4-1. Have you ever thought of using fractions in everyday activities like ordering pizza?

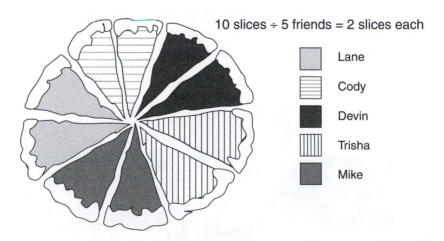

10 slices ÷ 5 friends = 2 slices each

Lane

Cody

Devin

Trisha

Mike

FIGURE 4-1 We use fractions daily, on such simple tasks as ordering pizza.

Objective

4.2 Explain advantages of using fractions.

As illustrated in the previous example, we utilize fractions in our everyday activities. Fractions help us to divide items into equal and unequal parts. For example, a pie may be divided into 6 equal slices.

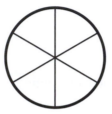

Alternately, one-half of the pie may be divided into three equal slices and the other half may be divided into four equal slices.

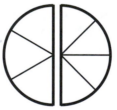

Regardless of how we decide to divide an item, fractions help to accomplish the task. See how many other items you can think of that we divide using fractions.

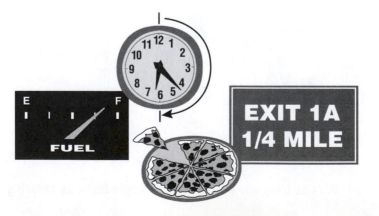

Objective

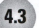 Find the numerator.

A **numerator** identifies the number of parts represented in the fraction. It is shown as the top number in the fraction.

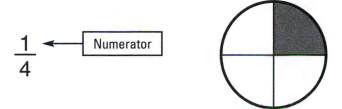

$$\frac{1}{4} \longleftarrow \boxed{\text{Numerator}}$$

SKILL SHARPENER

Circle the numerator in the following fractions.

1. $\frac{1}{2}$ 6. $\frac{12}{15}$

2. $\frac{4}{5}$ 7. $\frac{3}{4}$

3. $\frac{12}{32}$ 8. $\frac{8}{12}$

4. $\frac{6}{7}$ 9. $\frac{10}{12}$

5. $\frac{9}{10}$ 10. $\frac{5}{9}$

Objective

4.4 Find the denominator.

A **denominator** represents the number of parts into which an item is divided. For example, if the number below the line (denominator) is 2, the item is divided into 2 equal parts. If the denominator is 12, the item is divided into 12 equal parts.

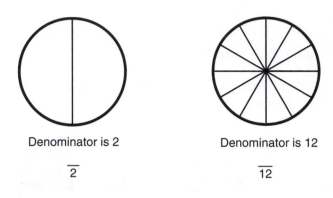

Denominator is 2   Denominator is 12

$$\overline{2}$$ $$\overline{12}$$

SKILL SHARPENER

Circle the denominator in the following fractions.

1. $\frac{3}{4}$ 6. $\frac{4}{7}$

2. $\frac{9}{16}$ 7. $\frac{3}{8}$

3. $\frac{1}{2}$ 8. $\frac{9}{16}$

4. $\frac{5}{8}$ 9. $\frac{22}{100}$

5. $\frac{17}{32}$ 10. $\frac{56}{9}$

Objective

4.5 Order fractions.

It is important to understand the value of fractions. Since the value of a fraction depends on both the numerator and denominator, you must consider both when determining the value of a fraction. Later, you will learn to find common denominators of fractions. This will make it easy to order fractions. For now, however, a simpler approach will help you begin to visualize fractions as part of a whole, rather than just a number on paper.

Example

Order the following fractions from lowest to highest, using the graphic representation of a pie to assist you. You may choose, instead, to convert each fraction to a decimal by dividing the numerator by the denominator. Then compare the decimals as demonstrated in Objective 5.3.

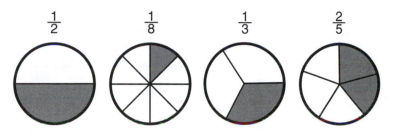

Compare the fractions using the graphic representation of the pies.

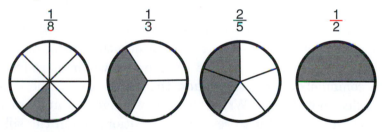

Order the following fractions from smallest to largest.

1. $\frac{2}{3}$ $\frac{5}{8}$ $\frac{2}{5}$ _____

2. $\frac{2}{8}$ $\frac{1}{5}$ $\frac{6}{8}$ _____

3. $\frac{1}{2}$ $\frac{3}{4}$ $\frac{1}{5}$ _____

4. $\frac{1}{3}$ $\frac{2}{3}$ $\frac{1}{5}$ _____

5. $\frac{3}{6}$ $\frac{2}{3}$ $\frac{1}{5}$ _____

6. $\frac{3}{8}$ $\frac{1}{4}$ $\frac{1}{8}$ _____

7. $\frac{2}{6}$ $\frac{2}{3}$ $\frac{1}{8}$ _____

8. $\frac{4}{5}$ $\frac{3}{9}$ $\frac{2}{3}$ _____

9. $\frac{6}{7}$ $\frac{8}{9}$ $\frac{7}{8}$ _____

10. $\frac{1}{2}$ $\frac{5}{6}$ $\frac{3}{4}$ _____

Objective

4.6 Add fractions with common denominators.

There are times when fractions must be added. This is easily done when the fractions share **common denominators** or denominators that are the same. To find the sum of two or more fractions with common denominators, add the numerators. The denominator does not change. Write the sum of the numerators over the common denominator to reveal the solution. When the solution reveals an improper fraction, convert to a proper fraction or mixed number as illustrated in Objective 4.17.

The problem:

$$\frac{1}{8} + \frac{3}{8} = \underline{\quad}$$

Set up as:

$$\frac{1}{8} + \frac{3}{8} = \underline{\quad}$$

Add.

$$\frac{1+3}{8} = \frac{4}{8}$$

Solution: $\frac{1}{8} + \frac{3}{8} = \frac{4}{8}$

SKILL SHARPENER

Add the following fractions.

1. $\frac{4}{5} + \frac{3}{5} =$ _____

2. $\frac{2}{3} + \frac{2}{3} =$ _____

3. $\frac{12}{16} + \frac{2}{16} =$ _____

4. $\frac{2}{6} + \frac{1}{6} =$ _____

5. $\frac{2}{9} + \frac{3}{9} =$ _____

6. $\frac{3}{8} + \frac{1}{8} =$ _____

7. $\frac{7}{8} + \frac{2}{8} =$ _____

8. $\frac{1}{7} + \frac{3}{7} =$ _____

9. $\frac{12}{50} + \frac{33}{50} =$ _____

10. $\frac{2}{25} + \frac{22}{25} =$ _____

Objective

4.7 Subtract fractions with common denominators.

To subtract fractions that share a common denominator, simply subtract the numerators. The denominator does not change. When solutions contain improper fractions, convert to proper fractions or mixed numbers as illustrated in Objective 4.17.

56

The problem:

$$\frac{9}{16} - \frac{3}{16} = \underline{\qquad}$$

Set up as:

$$\frac{9}{16} - \frac{3}{16} = \underline{\qquad}$$

Subtract.

$$\frac{9}{16} - \frac{3}{16} = \frac{6}{16}$$

Solution: $\frac{9}{16} - \frac{3}{16} = \frac{6}{16}$

SKILL SHARPENER

Subtract the following fractions.

1. $\frac{3}{4} - \frac{1}{4} =$ _____

2. $\frac{9}{18} - \frac{3}{18} =$ _____

3. $\frac{2}{3} - \frac{1}{3} =$ _____

4. $\frac{9}{12} - \frac{4}{12} =$ _____

5. $\frac{40}{50} - \frac{13}{50} =$ _____

6. $\frac{12}{16} - \frac{3}{16} =$ _____

7. $\frac{24}{100} - \frac{6}{100} =$ _____

8. $\frac{7}{80} - \frac{2}{80} =$ _____

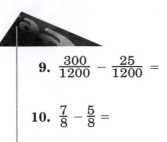

9. $\dfrac{300}{1200} - \dfrac{25}{1200} =$ _____

10. $\dfrac{7}{8} - \dfrac{5}{8} =$ _____

Objective

4.8 Define mixed number.

A **mixed number** is a combination of a whole number and a fraction. As you will see, it is sometimes necessary to convert mixed numbers to improper fractions.

Objective

4.9 Add mixed numbers with common denominators.

To add mixed numbers with common denominators, first add the numerators of the fractions. The denominator will not change. If the sum of the numerators is greater than the denominator, convert the fraction to a mixed number. Then add the whole numbers and, if applicable, add the whole number of the mixed number.

The problem:

$$1\tfrac{1}{3} + 2\tfrac{1}{3} = \underline{\quad\quad}$$

Set up as:

$$1\tfrac{1}{3} + 2\tfrac{1}{3} = \underline{\quad\quad}$$

Add fractions.

$$\tfrac{1}{3} + \tfrac{1}{3} = \tfrac{2}{3}$$

Add whole numbers.

$$1 + 2 = 3$$

Combine.

$$3\frac{2}{3}$$

Solution: $1\frac{1}{3} + 2\frac{1}{3} = 3\frac{2}{3}$

SKILL SHARPENER

Add the following fractions.

1. $1\frac{2}{5} + 2\frac{1}{5} =$ _____

2. $2\frac{6}{9} + 1\frac{1}{9} =$ _____

3. $5\frac{1}{12} + 1\frac{5}{12} =$ _____

4. $3\frac{2}{8} + 1\frac{5}{8} =$ _____

5. $1\frac{13}{50} + 2\frac{2}{50} =$ _____

6. $2\frac{3}{24} + 1\frac{6}{24} =$ _____

7. $4\frac{5}{8} + 3\frac{1}{8} =$ _____

8. $1\frac{3}{7} + 2\frac{1}{7} =$ _____

9. $2\frac{1}{20} + 1\frac{1}{20} =$ _____

10. $3\frac{15}{16} + 1\frac{2}{16} =$ _____

Objective

4.10 Subtract mixed numbers with common denominators.

When subtracting mixed numbers with common denominators, first subtract the numerators of the fractions. If necessary, you may borrow from the whole number. Then subtract the whole numbers. The combination of the differences is your solution. You may also convert the mixed numbers to improper fractions as explained in Objective 4.24. Then subtract and convert the difference to a proper fraction or mixed number.

The problem:

$$3\frac{9}{16} - 1\frac{4}{16} = \underline{\hspace{1cm}}$$

Set up as:

$$3\frac{9}{16} - 1\frac{4}{16} = \underline{\hspace{1cm}}$$

Subtract fractions.

$$\frac{9}{16} - \frac{4}{16} = \frac{5}{16}$$

Subtract whole numbers.

$$3 - 1 = 2$$

Combine.

$$2\frac{5}{16}$$

Solution: $3\frac{9}{16} - 1\frac{4}{16} = 2\frac{5}{16}$

SKILL SHARPENER

Find the difference.

1. $1\frac{3}{4} - \frac{1}{4} =$ _____

2. $5\frac{5}{6} - 1\frac{2}{6} =$ _____

3. $3\frac{5}{24} - 1\frac{3}{24} =$ _____

4. $2\frac{6}{8} - 1\frac{1}{8} =$ _____

5. $1\frac{9}{10} - \frac{3}{10} =$ _____

6. $11\frac{15}{16} - 5\frac{1}{16} =$ _____

7. $3\frac{4}{9} - 1\frac{1}{9} =$ _____

8. $3\frac{4}{11} - 1\frac{3}{11} =$ _____

9. $5\frac{15}{16} - 2\frac{12}{16} =$ _____

10. $9\frac{30}{100} - 6\frac{10}{100} =$ _____

Objective

4.11 Define factors.

Factors are pairs of numbers that, when multiplied, form a certain product. Factors of a number are found by using multiplication to determine every combination of that number.

Example

To find the factors of 16, determine every possible combination of 16 using multiplication.

$1 \times 16 = 16$	Factors of 16 are
$2 \times 8 = 16$	1, 2, 4, 8, and 16.
$4 \times 4 = 16$	

Later, this skill will be used to perform other operations.

Find the factors of the following numbers.

1. 8 _____

2. 9 _____

3. 12 _____

4. 18 _____

5. 24 _____

6. 20 _____

7. 10 _____

8. 6 _____

9. 14 _____

10. 22 _____

Objective

4.12 Find common factors.

A **common factor** is a factor that belongs to two or more numbers. To find the common factor(s) of two numbers, first find the factors for each number.

The problem:

Find factors of 8 and 12.

Find all the ways you can multiply to produce 8 and 12.

8	12
$1 \times 8 = 8$	$1 \times 12 = 12$
$2 \times 4 = 8$	$2 \times 6 = 12$
	$3 \times 4 = 12$

Now find the common factors.

8	12
$1 \times 8 = 8$	$1 \times 12 = 12$
$2 \times 4 = 8$	$2 \times 6 = 12$
	$3 \times 4 = 12$

Solution: Common factors of 8 and 12 are 1, 2, and 4.

The factors common to both numbers are common factors. Common factors in this set are 1, 2, and 4. Factors uncommon to a set of numbers are **uncommon factors**. The uncommon factors in this set are 3, 6, 8, and 12.

SKILL SHARPENER

Find common factors for the following sets of numbers.

1. 12, 16 _____

2. 8, 12 _____

3. 10, 15 _____

4. 24, 12 _____

5. 3, 8 _____

6. 5, 12 _____

7. 6, 9, 12 _____

8. 16, 8, 24 _____

9. 18, 6, 9 _____

10. 9, 36, 6 _____

Objective

4.13 Find the greatest common factor.

The **greatest common factor (GCF)** is the largest factor that two or more numbers have in common. To find the greatest common factor, first find the common factors. Then find the largest factor that the two numbers have in common. This is the greatest common factor.

In the earlier example, we found that common factors for 8 and 12 are 1, 2, and 4. Therefore, the greatest common factor for 8 and 12 is 4.

Find the greatest common factor for the following sets of numbers.

1. 6, 9 _____

2. 12, 20 _____

3. 3, 12 _____

4. 9, 6 _____

5. 2, 3, 9 _____

6. 12, 24 _____

7. 5, 12 _____

8. 4, 12, 9 _____

9. 3, 5, 9 _____

10. 15, 3, 5 _____

Objective

4.14 Reduce fractions.

To make fractions clearer, reduce them to their lowest terms by finding the greatest common factor of the numerator and denominator. Divide both the numerator and denominator by their greatest common factor. The result is a reduced fraction.

To reduce $\frac{4}{6}$ to its lowest terms:

Find the factors of the numerator and denominator.

4	6
$1 \times 4 = 4$	$1 \times 6 = 6$
$2 \times 2 = 4$	$2 \times 3 = 6$

Find the GCF.

The GCF is 2.

Divide the numerator and denominator by the GCF to reduce the fraction to its lowest terms.

$$\frac{4 \div 2}{6 \div 2} = \frac{2}{3}$$

SKILL SHARPENER

Reduce the following fractions to their lowest terms.

1. $\frac{6}{8}$ _____

2. $\frac{5}{25}$ _____

3. $\frac{9}{81}$ _____

4. $\frac{6}{9}$ _____

5. $\frac{3}{6}$ _____

6. $\frac{2}{8}$ _____

7. $\frac{10}{20}$ _____

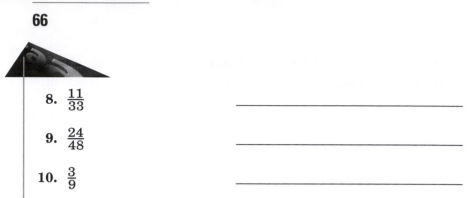

8. $\frac{11}{33}$ _____

9. $\frac{24}{48}$ _____

10. $\frac{3}{9}$ _____

Objective

4.15 Define proper fraction.

A **proper fraction** is one in which the denominator is greater than the numerator.

Proper fraction:

$\frac{9}{16}$ | Numerator (**smaller**)
| Denominator (**larger**)

SKILL SHARPENER

Determine if the following fractions are proper by placing **P** beside those that are proper and **I** (for improper) beside those that are not proper.

1. $\frac{3}{8}$ _____

2. $\frac{7}{16}$ _____

3. $\frac{9}{8}$ _____

4. $\frac{4}{3}$ _____

5. $\frac{12}{15}$ _____

6. $\frac{11}{16}$ _____

7. $\frac{90}{12}$ _____

8. $\frac{33}{2}$ _____

9. $\frac{12}{45}$ _____

10. $\frac{1}{25}$ _____

Objective

 Define improper fraction.

An **improper fraction** is one in which the numerator is greater than the denominator. Improper fractions may be changed to proper fractions or mixed numbers to make them easier to read.

Improper fraction:

$\dfrac{12}{10}$

| Numerator (**larger**) |
| Denominator (**smaller**) |

SKILL SHARPENER

Place **P** beside the following fractions that are proper and **I** next to those that are improper.

1. $\dfrac{2}{4}$ _____

2. $\dfrac{9}{6}$ _____

3. $\dfrac{5}{4}$ _____

4. $\dfrac{15}{16}$ _____

5. $\dfrac{6}{9}$ _____

6. $\dfrac{12}{3}$ _____

7. $\dfrac{4}{8}$ _____

8. $\dfrac{2}{3}$ _____

9. $\dfrac{10}{2}$ _____

10. $\dfrac{6}{5}$ _____

Objective

4.17 Change improper fractions to proper fractions.

To change improper fractions to proper fractions, divide the denominator into the numerator. The result is a proper fraction that may or may not need to be reduced.

The problem:

Convert the improper fraction $\frac{23}{16}$ to a proper fraction.

Divide the denominator into the numerator.

$$23 \div 16 = \underline{}$$

Set up as:

$$16 \overline{\smash{\big)}\,23}$$

Divide.

$$16 \overline{\smash{\big)}\,\begin{array}{c} 1 \\ 23 \end{array}}$$
$$\underline{16}$$
$$7$$

Solution: $1\frac{7}{16}$

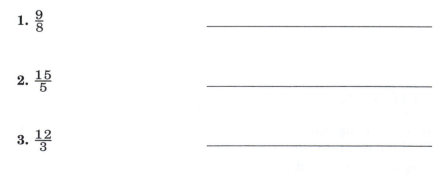

SKILL SHARPENER

Change the following improper fractions to proper fractions or mixed numbers.

1. $\frac{9}{8}$ _____

2. $\frac{15}{5}$ _____

3. $\frac{12}{3}$ _____

4. $\frac{12}{7}$ _____

5. $\frac{6}{4}$ _____

6. $\frac{6}{3}$ _____

7. $\frac{8}{2}$ _____

8. $\frac{15}{4}$ _____

9. $\frac{19}{3}$ _____

10. $\frac{22}{12}$ _____

Objective

4.18 Define multiple.

A **multiple** of a number is the product of a whole number and another whole number.

Example

Multiples of **2** are 2, 4, 6, 8, 10, 12, 14, 16, 18, 20, 22, 24, and so on.

Multiples of **3** are 3, 6, 9, 12, 15, 18, 21, 24, 27, 30, 33, 36, and so on.

SKILL SHARPENER

List some multiples of each of the following numbers.

1. 4 _____

2. 5 _____

3. 6 _____

4. 7 _____

5. 8 _____

Objective

4.19 Define least common multiple.

The **least common multiple** is the smallest multiple that is shared by two or more numbers.

Example

Multiples of **2** are 2, 4, 6, 8, 10, 12, 14, 16, 18, 20, 22, 24, and so on.

Multiples of **3** are 3, 6, 9, 12, 15, 18, 21, 24, 27, 30, 33, 36, and so on.

Common multiples of **2** and **3** are 6, 12, 18, 24.

The least common multiple is 6.

SKILL SHARPENER

Find the least common multiples of the following.

1. 2, 4 _____

2. 3, 6 _____

3. 4, 5 _____

4. 12, 3 _____

5. 7, 2 _____

6. 8, 3 _____

7. 9, 2 _____

8. 10, 20, 4 _____

9. 9, 12, 4 _____

10. 2, 6, 8 _____

Objective

4.20 Find the least common denominator.

The **least common denominator (LCD)** is the lowest number into which all the denominators in a set can be divided. To find the least common denominator, find the least common multiple of each of the denominators in the set.

The problem:

Find the least common denominator of $\frac{1}{4}$, $\frac{1}{3}$, and $\frac{1}{6}$.

Find the multiples of each denominator.

4, 8, 12, 16, 20, 24, and so on.

3, 6, 9, 12, 15, 18, 21, and so on.

6, 12, 18, 24, 30, and so on.

Find least common multiple (LCM).

4, 8, **12**, 16, 20, 24, and so on.

LCM ← 3, 6, 9, **12**, 15, 18, 21, and so on.

6, **12**, 18, 24, 30, and so on.

Solution: The least common multiple is 12; therefore, the LCD is 12.

SKILL SHARPENER

Find the least common denominator for each of the following sets of fractions.

1. $\frac{2}{3}$ $\frac{5}{6}$ _____

2. $\frac{1}{2}$ $\frac{3}{4}$ _____

3. $\frac{7}{8}$ $\frac{7}{16}$ _____

4. $\frac{3}{4}$ $\frac{4}{5}$ _____

5. $\frac{8}{10}$ $\frac{12}{20}$ _____

6. $\frac{3}{8}$ $\frac{7}{16}$ _____

7. $\frac{7}{8}$ $\frac{1}{4}$ $\frac{2}{3}$ _____

8. $\frac{4}{5}$ $\frac{3}{10}$ _____

9. $\frac{2}{3}$ $\frac{3}{4}$ $\frac{4}{5}$ _____

10. $\frac{1}{2}$ $\frac{6}{8}$ $\frac{3}{4}$ _____

Objective

 Add fractions with uncommon denominators.

To add fractions with **uncommon denominators**, first find the least common denominator. Next, convert each fraction to a fraction utilizing the least common denominator. Then add the numerators and reduce as necessary.

The problem:

Add the following fractions with uncommon denominators:

$$\frac{3}{4} + \frac{1}{3} = \underline{\hspace{1cm}}$$

Find the LCM and the LCD.

4, 8, 12, 16, 20, and so on.

3, 6, 9, 12, 15, and so on.

The LCM is 12, so the LCD will be 12.

Now change the denominators in both fractions to the LCD.

$$\frac{3}{4} + \frac{1}{3} = \underline{\hspace{1cm}}$$

$$\frac{}{12} + \frac{}{12} = \underline{\hspace{1cm}}$$

Multiply each numerator by the number of times the original denominators go into the LCD.

$$\frac{3}{4} + \frac{1}{3}$$

| $4 \times 3 = 12$ | $\times 3$ | | $\times 4$ | $3 \times 4 = 12$ |

$$\frac{}{12} + \frac{}{12}$$

Now multiply the original numerators by the shaded factors to determine new numerators.

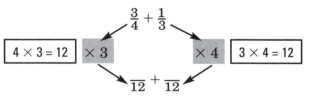

| $3 \times 3 = 9$ | $\rightarrow$ | $\frac{9}{12} + \frac{4}{12}$ | $\leftarrow$ | $1 \times 4 = 4$ |

Add.

$$\frac{9}{12} + \frac{4}{12} = \frac{13}{12}$$

Solution: $\frac{3}{4} + \frac{1}{3} = \frac{13}{12}$ or $1\frac{1}{12}$

SKILL SHARPENER

Add the following fractions with uncommon denominators.

1. $\frac{1}{3} + \frac{2}{4} =$ _____

2. $\frac{2}{3} + \frac{1}{2} =$ _____

3. $\frac{3}{4} + \frac{7}{8} =$ _____

4. $\frac{1}{2} + \frac{3}{8} =$ _____

5. $\frac{3}{9} + \frac{2}{3} =$ _____

6. $\frac{4}{5} + \frac{5}{6} =$ _____

7. $\frac{1}{4} + \frac{1}{16} =$ _____

8. $\frac{2}{5} + \frac{6}{10} =$ _____

9. $\frac{3}{8} + \frac{9}{16} =$ _____

10. $\frac{3}{10} + \frac{19}{20} + \frac{3}{5} =$ _____

Objective

4.22 Subtract fractions with uncommon denominators.

To subtract fractions with uncommon denominators, find the least common denominator. Next, convert each fraction to a fraction utilizing the least common denominator. Then subtract the numerators and reduce as necessary.

The problem:

$$\frac{1}{2} - \frac{1}{16} = \underline{\qquad}$$

Find the LCM, which will also be the LCD.

2, 4, 6, 8, 10, 12, 14, 16, and so on.

16, 32, 48, 64, and so on.

Solution: The LCM is 16; therefore, the LCD is 16.

Now change the denominators in both fractions to the LCD.

$$\frac{1}{2} - \frac{1}{16} = \underline{\qquad}$$

$$\overline{16} - \overline{16} = \underline{\qquad}$$

Multiply each numerator by the number of times the original denominators go into the LCD.

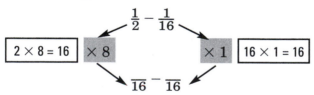

Now multiply the original numerators by the shaded factors.

$$\boxed{1 \times 8 = 8} \longrightarrow \frac{8}{16} - \frac{1}{16} \longleftarrow \boxed{1 \times 1 = 1}$$

Subtract.

$$\frac{8}{16} - \frac{1}{16} = \frac{7}{16}$$

Solution: $\frac{1}{2} - \frac{1}{16} = \frac{7}{16}$

SKILL SHARPENER

Subtract the following fractions with uncommon denominators.

1. $\frac{2}{3} - \frac{1}{4} =$ _____

2. $\frac{12}{16} - \frac{1}{2} =$ _____

3. $\frac{4}{5} - \frac{1}{3} =$ _____

4. $\frac{7}{8} - \frac{3}{5} =$ _____

5. $\frac{9}{10} - \frac{2}{5} =$ _____

6. $\frac{3}{4} - \frac{1}{2} =$ _____

7. $\frac{9}{18} - \frac{1}{3} =$ _____

8. $\frac{8}{9} - \frac{3}{7} =$ _____

9. $\frac{5}{9} - \frac{3}{8} =$ _____

10. $\frac{7}{11} - \frac{1}{22} =$ _____

Objective

4.23 Use borrowing to subtract fractions.

When subtracting mixed numbers, it is sometimes necessary to borrow. If fractions have uncommon denominators, find the least common denominator before subtracting.

The problem:

$$5\frac{1}{3} - 2\frac{2}{3} = \underline{\hspace{1cm}}$$

Subtract fractions.

$$\frac{1}{3} - \frac{2}{3} = \underline{\hspace{1cm}}$$

Since you cannot subtract 2 from 1, you will have to borrow from the whole number 5.

$$\cancel{5}\frac{1}{3} - 2\frac{2}{3}$$
$$\downarrow$$
$$4\frac{4}{3} - 2\frac{2}{3}$$

Now subtract the fractions.

$$\frac{4}{3} - \frac{2}{3} = \frac{2}{3}$$

Subtract the whole numbers.

$$4 - 2 = 2$$

Combine.

$$2\frac{2}{3}$$

Solution: $5\frac{1}{3} - 2\frac{2}{3} = 2\frac{2}{3}$

Note: An alternate way to subtract this is to convert to improper fractions.

$$5\frac{1}{3} - 2\frac{2}{3} = \underline{\hspace{1cm}}$$

To convert, multiply the denominator by the whole number and add the numerator.

$$(3 \times 5) + 1 - (3 \times 2) + 2$$

$$15 + 1 \quad - \quad 6 + 2$$

$$\frac{16}{3} \quad - \quad \frac{8}{3} = \frac{8}{3}$$

Now convert back to a proper fraction by dividing the numerator by the denominator.

$$8 \div 3 = \underline{\hspace{1.5cm}}$$

$$\begin{array}{r} 2 \\ 3\overline{)8} \\ \underline{6} \\ 2 \end{array}$$

Solution: $5\frac{1}{3} - 2\frac{2}{3} = 2\frac{2}{3}$

Now practice by solving this problem in which the denominators are different.

$$4\frac{1}{4} - 2\frac{3}{8} = \underline{\hspace{1.5cm}}$$

The problem: Subtract the following fractions with uncommon denominators:

$$4\frac{1}{4} - 2\frac{3}{8} = \underline{\hspace{1.5cm}}$$

Find the LCM and LCD.

4, 8, 12, 16, 20, and so on.

8, 16, 24, 32, 40, and so on.

Now change the denominators in both fractions to the LCD.

$$4\frac{1}{4} - 2\frac{3}{8} = \underline{\hspace{1.5cm}}$$

$$\frac{}{8} - \frac{}{8} = \underline{\hspace{1.5cm}}$$

Multiply each numerator by the number of times the original denominator goes into the LCD.

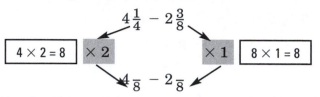

Now multiply the original numerators by the shaded factors.

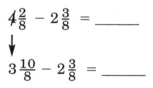

Subtract.

$$4\tfrac{2}{8} - 2\tfrac{3}{8} = \underline{\hspace{1.5cm}}$$

Borrow.

$$4\tfrac{2}{8} - 2\tfrac{3}{8} = \underline{\hspace{1.5cm}}$$

$$\downarrow$$

$$3\tfrac{10}{8} - 2\tfrac{3}{8} = \underline{\hspace{1.5cm}}$$

Subtract fractions.

$$\tfrac{10}{8} - \tfrac{3}{8} = \tfrac{7}{8}$$

Subtract whole numbers.

$$3 - 2 = 1$$

Combine.

$$1\tfrac{7}{8}$$

Solution: $4\tfrac{1}{4} - 2\tfrac{3}{8} = 1\tfrac{7}{8}$

Now figure this problem by converting to improper fractions. The result should be the same.

SKILL SHARPENER

Subtract the following fractions.

1. $4\frac{5}{7} - 1\frac{1}{7} =$ _____

2. $3\frac{1}{2} - 1\frac{1}{2} =$ _____

3. $7\frac{3}{4} - 3\frac{1}{4} =$ _____

4. $4\frac{3}{8} - \frac{1}{8} =$ _____

5. $3\frac{15}{16}$ $-1\frac{5}{16}$

6. $4\frac{3}{4}$ $-2\frac{7}{8}$

7. $5\frac{1}{2}$ $-2\frac{7}{8}$

8. $6\frac{7}{8}$ $-\frac{11}{12}$

9. $2\frac{3}{5}$ $-1\frac{5}{8}$

10. $1\frac{2}{3}$ $-\frac{9}{11}$

Objective

4.24 Change mixed numbers to improper fractions.

To change a mixed number to an improper fraction, multiply the denominator by the whole number and add the numerator. This is your new numerator. The denominator stays the same.

The problem:

Change $4\frac{3}{8}$ to an improper fraction.

Multiply the whole number and denominator.

$$4 \times 8 = 32$$

Add the numerator.

$$32 + 3 = 35$$

This is the new numerator. The denominator does not change.

Solution: $4\frac{3}{8} = \frac{35}{8}$

Note: Another way to set up the equation is:

(whole number $\times$ denominator) $+$ numerator $=$ _____

(4 $\times$ 8) $+$ 3 $=$ _____

32                              $+$ 3 $=$ 35

SKILL SHARPENER

Change these mixed numbers to improper fractions.

1. $3\frac{2}{9}$ _____

2. $8\frac{5}{8}$ _____

3. $2\frac{3}{4}$ _____

4. $7\frac{2}{6}$ _____

5. $1\frac{3}{11}$ _____

6. $9\frac{34}{50}$ _____

7. $6\frac{9}{12}$ _____

8. $5\frac{5}{9}$ _____

9. $12\frac{6}{10}$ _____

10. $3\frac{1}{2}$ _____

Objective

4.25 Multiply fractions.

To multiply simple fractions, find the product of the numerators and the product of the denominators. Reduce if necessary.

The problem:

$$\frac{1}{3} \times \frac{2}{3} = \underline{\hspace{2cm}}$$

Set up as:

$$\frac{1 \times 2 =}{3 \times 3 =}$$

Multiply:

$$\frac{1 \times 2 = 2}{3 \times 3 = 9}$$

Solution: $\frac{1}{3} \times \frac{2}{3} = \frac{2}{9}$

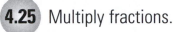
SKILL SHARPENER

Find the products of the following fractions.

1. $\frac{2}{3} \times \frac{3}{4} =$ _____

2. $\frac{1}{8} \times \frac{2}{3} =$ _____

3. $\frac{4}{5} \times \frac{7}{8} =$ _____

4. $\frac{1}{2} \times \frac{5}{9} =$ _____

5. $\frac{2}{6} \times \frac{3}{4} =$ _____

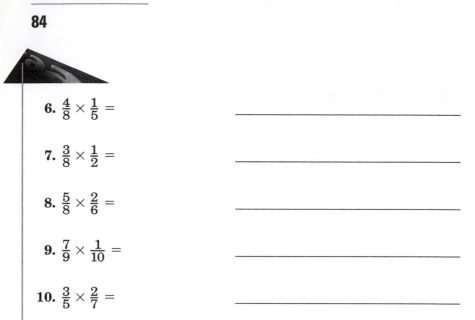

6. $\frac{4}{8} \times \frac{1}{5} =$ _____

7. $\frac{3}{8} \times \frac{1}{2} =$ _____

8. $\frac{5}{8} \times \frac{2}{6} =$ _____

9. $\frac{7}{9} \times \frac{1}{10} =$ _____

10. $\frac{3}{5} \times \frac{2}{7} =$ _____

Objective

4.26 Multiply fractions using canceling.

To utilize **canceling** to find the product of two fractions, set the equation up as follows.

The problem:
$$\frac{3}{8} \times \frac{4}{12} = \text{\_\_\_\_}$$

Cancel by determining if any numerator or denominator is divisible by another.
$$\frac{3}{8} \times \frac{4}{12} = \text{\_\_\_\_}$$

Since 4 goes into 8 twice, replace the 8 with 2 and the 4 with 1:
$$\frac{3}{_2\cancel{8}} \times \frac{\cancel{4}^1}{12}$$

Since 3 goes into 12 four times, cancel the 3 and write 1 and replace the 12 with 4:
$$\frac{^1\cancel{3}}{2} \times \frac{1}{\cancel{12}_4}$$

We now have:

$$\frac{1}{2} \times \frac{1}{4} = \underline{\hspace{2cm}}$$

Multiply.

$$\frac{1 \times 1 = 1}{2 \times 4 = 8}$$

Solution: $\frac{3}{8} \times \frac{4}{12} = \frac{1}{8}$

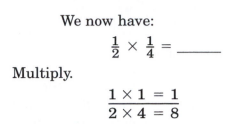

SKILL SHARPENER

Find the product using canceling.

1. $\frac{1}{6} \times \frac{2}{3} =$ _____

2. $\frac{3}{9} \times \frac{1}{3} =$ _____

3. $\frac{1}{2} \times \frac{4}{8} =$ _____

4. $\frac{3}{4} \times \frac{1}{6} =$ _____

5. $\frac{4}{7} \times \frac{5}{6} =$ _____

6. $\frac{3}{8} \times \frac{2}{6} =$ _____

7. $\frac{7}{9} \times \frac{3}{4} =$ _____

8. $\frac{5}{6} \times \frac{3}{4} =$ _____

9. $\frac{5}{15} \times \frac{1}{5} =$ _____

10. $\frac{4}{6} \times \frac{12}{16} =$ _____

Objective

 Multiply fractions and whole numbers.

When multiplying fractions and whole numbers, first convert the whole number to an improper fraction. Multiply numerators and denominators. Then convert back to a proper fraction or mixed number.

The problem:

$$3 \times \frac{1}{8} = \underline{\hspace{1.5cm}}$$

Convert the whole number to an improper fraction by using a denominator of 1.

$$\frac{3}{1} \times \frac{1}{8} = \underline{\hspace{1.5cm}}$$

Multiply the numerators and denominators.

$$\frac{3 \times 1 = 3}{1 \times 8 = 8}$$

Solution: $3 \times \frac{1}{8} = \frac{3}{8}$

SKILL SHARPENER

Find the products.

1. $\frac{2}{3} \times 12 =$ _____

2. $3 \times \frac{1}{5} =$ _____

3. $4 \times \frac{4}{5} =$ _____

4. $2 \times \frac{5}{6} =$ _____

5. $\frac{1}{2}$
$\times\ 10$

6. $\frac{1}{3}$
$\times\ 5$

7. $\frac{4}{6}$
$\times\ 9$

8. 3
$\times\ \frac{5}{9}$

9. 9
$\times\ \frac{5}{16}$

10. 5
$\times\ \frac{1}{9}$

Objective

4.28 Multiply fractions and mixed numbers.

To multiply a fraction with a mixed number, convert the mixed number to an improper fraction. Then multiply to find the product of the numerators and the product of the denominators. Reduce to lowest terms.

The problem:

$$\frac{1}{5} \times 2\frac{1}{2} = \underline{\qquad}$$

Convert the mixed number ($2\frac{1}{2}$) to an improper fraction.

Multiply the whole number by the denominator, then add the numerator.

(whole number $\times$ denominator) + numerator $=$ \underline{\qquad}

(2×2) $+$ 1 $=$ \underline{\qquad}

4 $+$ 1 $=$ 5

The new numerator is 5. The denominator stays the same.

$\frac{5}{2}$

Set up as:

$$\frac{1}{5} \times \frac{5}{2} = \underline{\hspace{2cm}}$$

Multiply the numerators and denominators. In this case, you may use canceling to change both 5s to 1s.

Multiply	**Cancel**
$\dfrac{1 \times 5 = 5}{5 \times 2 = 10}$	$\dfrac{1}{{}_1\cancel{5}} \times \dfrac{\cancel{5}^{\,1}}{2} = \dfrac{1}{2}$

If necessary, reduce by finding the LCF.*

$$\frac{5}{1 \times \boxed{5} = 5}$$

$$\frac{10}{\begin{array}{l} 1 \times 10 = 10 \\ 2 \times \boxed{5} = 10 \end{array}}$$

LCF is 5. Divide 5 into $\dfrac{5}{10}$.

$$\frac{5 \div 5 = 1}{10 \div 5 = 2}$$

Solution: $\dfrac{1}{5} \times 2\dfrac{1}{2} = \dfrac{1}{2}$

*By canceling, you eliminate one step (reducing).

SKILL SHARPENER

Find the product. Reduce to lowest terms.

1. $\dfrac{2}{3}$
    $\times\ 3\dfrac{1}{2}$

2. $\dfrac{3}{5}$
    $\times\ 2\dfrac{3}{4}$

3. $1\dfrac{3}{4}$
    $\times\ \dfrac{2}{5}$

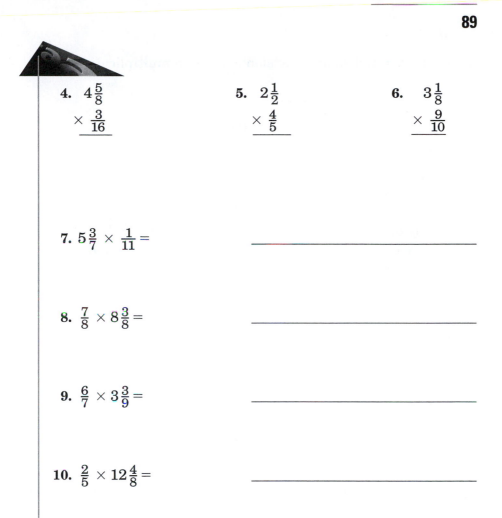

4. $4\frac{5}{8}$

$\times \frac{3}{16}$

5. $2\frac{1}{2}$

$\times \frac{4}{5}$

6. $3\frac{1}{8}$

$\times \frac{9}{10}$

7. $5\frac{3}{7} \times \frac{1}{11} =$ _____

8. $\frac{7}{8} \times 8\frac{3}{8} =$ _____

9. $\frac{6}{7} \times 3\frac{3}{9} =$ _____

10. $\frac{2}{5} \times 12\frac{4}{8} =$ _____

Objective

4.29 Divide fractions.

To divide fractions, convert any mixed numbers to improper fractions. Invert the divisor and multiply numerators and denominators.

The problem:

$$\frac{4}{9} \div \frac{1}{3} = \underline{\qquad}$$

Invert divisor and change division symbol to multiplication.

$$\frac{4}{9} \times \frac{3}{1} = \underline{\hspace{1.5cm}}$$

Multiply numerators and   **OR**   Multiply by
denominators.   canceling.

$$\frac{4 \times 3 = 12}{9 \times 1 = \ 9}$$ $$3\ \cancel{\frac{4}{9}} \times \frac{\cancel{3}\,1}{1}$$

Reduce by dividing the   Then multiply
product by the LCF.   numerators and
                                                 denominators.

$$3\ \cancel{\frac{4}{9}} \times \frac{\cancel{3}\,1}{1} = \frac{4}{3}$$

12	9
1 × 12 = 12	1 × 9 = 9
2 × 6 = 12	**3** × 3 = 9
3 × 4 = 12	

LCF is 3.

$$\frac{12 \div 3 = 4}{9 \div 3 = 3}$$

Convert to mixed number.

$$4 \div 3 = \underline{\hspace{1cm}}$$

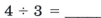

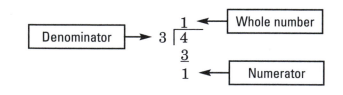

Solution: $\frac{4}{9} \div \frac{1}{3} = 1\frac{1}{3}$

SKILL SHARPENER

Divide the following fractions.

1. $\frac{3}{8} \div \frac{1}{4} =$ _____

2. $\frac{7}{8} \div \frac{2}{3} =$ _____

3. $\frac{16}{18} \div \frac{9}{12} =$ _____

4. $\frac{3}{4} \div \frac{1}{3} =$ _____

5. $\frac{2}{5} \overline{\smash{\big)}\, \frac{8}{10}}$ 6. $\frac{2}{3} \overline{\smash{\big)}\, 1\frac{3}{8}}$ 7. $\frac{1}{2} \overline{\smash{\big)}\, 3\frac{2}{5}}$

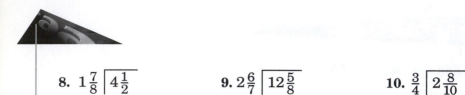

8. $1\frac{7}{8} \left) \overline{4\frac{1}{2}} \right.$

9. $2\frac{6}{7} \left) \overline{12\frac{5}{8}} \right.$

10. $\frac{3}{4} \left) \overline{2\frac{8}{10}} \right.$

CONCLUSION

Fractions are used in many ways in the health care industry. Medication dosages, heights and weights, and many other measurements use fractions. The ability to add, subtract, multiply, and divide fractions will help you to better perform as a health care provider, thus providing better care to your patients.

SELF-ASSESSMENT **POST-TEST**

Circle the numerator in the following fractions.

1. $\frac{1}{2}$

2. $\frac{23}{48}$

3. $\frac{2}{10}$

4. $\frac{6}{12}$

5. $\frac{125}{1,000}$

Circle the denominator in the following fractions.

6. $\frac{12}{14}$

7. $\frac{5}{61}$

8. $\frac{15}{16}$

9. $\frac{7}{8}$

10. $\frac{3}{4}$

Place the following fractions in order from smallest to largest.

11. $\frac{1}{2}$ $\frac{1}{3}$ $\frac{1}{4}$ $\frac{1}{5}$ $\frac{1}{6}$ _____

12. $\frac{7}{16}$ $\frac{3}{8}$ $\frac{1}{2}$ $\frac{9}{16}$ $\frac{3}{4}$ _____

13. $\frac{12}{15}$ $\frac{12}{16}$ $\frac{9}{10}$ $\frac{11}{16}$ $\frac{7}{8}$ _____

14. $\frac{6}{15}$ $\frac{4}{9}$ $\frac{10}{12}$ $\frac{3}{4}$ $\frac{4}{5}$ _____

15. $\frac{1}{2}$ $\frac{2}{3}$ $\frac{3}{4}$ $\frac{4}{5}$ $\frac{5}{6}$ _____

Add the following fractions with common denominators.

16. $\frac{1}{3} + \frac{2}{3} =$ _____

17. $\frac{3}{4} + \frac{1}{4} =$ _____

18. $\frac{15}{16} + \frac{2}{16} =$ _____

19. $\frac{3}{12} + \frac{2}{12} =$ _____

20. $\frac{6}{64} + \frac{12}{64} =$ _____

Subtract the following fractions with common denominators.

21. $\frac{12}{100} - \frac{10}{100} =$ _____

22. $\frac{98}{144} - \frac{62}{144} =$ _____

23. $\frac{9}{10} - \frac{6}{10} =$ _____

24. $\frac{3}{4} - \frac{1}{4} =$ _____

25. $\frac{4}{5} - \frac{2}{5} =$ _____

Add the following mixed numbers with common denominators.

26. $1\frac{2}{3} + 2\frac{1}{3} =$ _____

27. $1\frac{15}{16} + 2\frac{3}{16} =$ _____

28. $23\frac{1}{2} + 4\frac{1}{2} =$ _____

29. $12\frac{4}{5} + 6\frac{1}{5} =$ _____

30. $2\frac{1}{8} + 3\frac{3}{8} =$ _____

Subtract the following mixed numbers with common denominators.

31. $23\frac{1}{4} - 12\frac{3}{4} =$ _____

32. $56\frac{1}{4} - 2\frac{3}{4} =$ _____

33. $1\frac{15}{16} - 1\frac{2}{16} =$ _____

34. $39\frac{7}{8} - 3\frac{2}{8} =$ _____

35. $13\frac{2}{5} - 2\frac{3}{5} =$ _____

Find the factors for the following numbers.

36. 12 _____

37. 16 _____

38. 6 _____

39. 10 _____

40. 8 _____

Find the greatest common factor of the following pairs of numbers.

41. 12, 18 _____

42. 6, 12 _____

43. 9, 12 _____

44. 8, 16 _____

45. 12, 16 _____

96

Reduce the following fractions.

46. $\frac{9}{18}$ _____

47. $\frac{8}{24}$ _____

48. $\frac{2}{32}$ _____

49. $\frac{15}{45}$ _____

50. $\frac{21}{24}$ _____

Change the following improper fractions to proper fractions.

51. $\frac{10}{5}$ _____

52. $\frac{36}{9}$ _____

53. $\frac{7}{5}$ _____

54. $\frac{12}{3}$ _____

55. $\frac{45}{5}$ _____

Find least common multiples of the following sets of numbers.

56. 12, 4 _____

57. 9, 3 _____

58. 14, 2 _____

59. 20, 4 _____

60. 2, 10 _____

Find the least common denominator in the following sets of fractions.

61. $\frac{1}{4}$, $\frac{1}{6}$ _____

62. $\frac{3}{12}$, $\frac{4}{16}$ _____

63. $\frac{2}{3}$, $\frac{4}{8}$ _____

64. $\frac{15}{16}$, $\frac{2}{3}$ _____

65. $\frac{3}{4}$, $\frac{4}{5}$ _____

Add the following fractions with uncommon denominators.

66. $\frac{3}{12} + \frac{2}{3} =$ _____

67. $\frac{3}{4} + \frac{6}{8} =$ _____

68. $\frac{1}{2} + \frac{6}{7} =$ _____

69. $\frac{4}{5} + \frac{1}{3} =$ _____

70. $\frac{3}{8} + \frac{7}{16} =$ _____

Subtract the following fractions with uncommon denominators.

71. $\frac{2}{3} - \frac{1}{8} =$ _____

72. $\frac{5}{6} - \frac{3}{8} =$ _____

73. $\frac{1}{2} - \frac{1}{3} =$ _____

74. $\frac{3}{4} - \frac{1}{6} =$ _____

75. $\frac{7}{16} - \frac{8}{32} =$ _____

Subtract the following using borrowing.

76. $2 - \frac{2}{8} =$ _____

77. $4\frac{1}{3} - \frac{2}{3} =$ _____

78. $2\frac{1}{16} - 1\frac{3}{16} =$ _____

79. $4\frac{1}{5} - \frac{4}{5} =$ _____

80. $3\frac{6}{8} - 1\frac{7}{8} =$ _____

Change the following mixed numbers to improper fractions.

81. $1\frac{1}{8}$ _____

82. $3\frac{6}{9}$ _____

83. $3\frac{1}{2}$ _____

84. $12\frac{3}{4}$ _____

85. $2\frac{5}{8}$ _____

Find the product of each of the following.

86. $\frac{3}{4} \times \frac{2}{3} =$ _____

87. $\frac{1}{2} \times \frac{5}{6} =$ _____

88. $\frac{3}{8} \times \frac{4}{5} =$ _____

89. $\frac{5}{9} \times \frac{3}{4} =$ _____

90. $\frac{12}{16} \times \frac{7}{8} =$ _____

91. $\frac{2}{5} \times \frac{7}{8} =$ _____

92. $\frac{1}{4} \times \frac{8}{9} =$ _____

93. $\frac{2}{3} \times \frac{6}{18} =$ _____

94. $\frac{4}{5} \times \frac{7}{8} =$ _____

95. $\frac{2}{3} \times \frac{9}{8} =$ _____

Find the quotient for each of the following.

96. $\frac{12}{16} \div \frac{2}{3} =$ _____

97. $\frac{1}{2} \div \frac{1}{3} =$ _____

98. $\frac{5}{6} \div \frac{7}{16} =$ _____

99. $\frac{3}{8} \div \frac{1}{5} =$ _____

100. $\frac{7}{8} \div \frac{2}{3} =$ _____

Ratios and Proportions

LEARNING **OBJECTIVES**

After completing this chapter, the reader will be able to:

5.1 Define ratio.

5.2 Define proportion.

5.3 Determine if proportions are equal.

5.4 Solve for a missing component in a proportion.

5.5 Solve practical problems using proportions.

KEY **TERMS**

- extremes
- means
- proportion
- ratio
- terms

INTRODUCTION

Ratios and proportions are commonly used in health care and medicine to compare measurements. Many health care providers utilize ratios and proportions on a daily basis to solve a variety of equations and make comparisons between unlike items.

Objective

 Define ratio.

As you have already learned, we can compare quantities in different ways. A **ratio** is a comparison of numbers by division. The numbers that are compared are called the **terms**, or components, of the ratio. For example, we can compare the number of gray stethoscopes to the number of black stethoscopes in Figure 5-1.

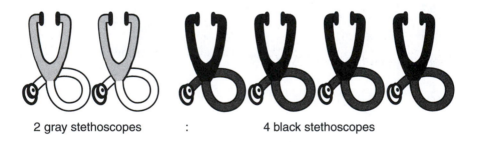

2 gray stethoscopes   :   4 black stethoscopes

FIGURE 5-1 This ratio is expressed as 2:4.

There are two gray stethoscopes and four black stethoscopes. Therefore, the ratio is 2 to 4, which may also be expressed as 2:4 or 2/4.

There is another way to express this ratio by reducing to the lowest common denominator. The ratio of 1 to 2 is also correct. For every one gray stethoscope, there are two black stethoscopes. Generally speaking, reducing to the LCD is helpful, especially when dealing with large numbers. Ratios are helpful in that they allow you to compare both like measurements and unlike measurements.

Consider the following examples.

Example A

On the day shift in the local hospital, there are two physical therapists and six physical therapy assistants on duty. What is the ratio of physical therapists to physical therapy assistants? Are these measurements alike or unlike?

If you answered 1:3 or 2:6 you are correct. And, of course, a physical therapist is unlike a physical therapy assistant (though the two are both measured as people). This ratio, or comparison, made it simple to measure the comparison between the two.

Example B

As you have likely learned, 1 pound is equal to 2.2 kg. State the ratio involved. Are these measurements alike or unlike?

If you answered 1:2.2 you are correct. Again, the measurements are unlike in that you are comparing pounds to kilograms.

Objective

5.2 Define proportion.

A **proportion** is an equation that states that two ratios are equal. Proportions are set up as 1:2::2:4. This is read: 1 is to 2 as 2 is to 4. The middle components of the proportion are called the **means** and the end, or outside, components are called **extremes**.

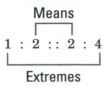

Objective

5.3 Determine if proportions are equal.

Comparing the product of the means to the product of the extremes determines if a proportion is equal. If the product of the means is equal to the product of the extremes, the proportion is said to be equal.

The problem: Determine if the proportion is equal:

$$1:2::2:4$$

Find the product of the means and the extremes.

Multiply the means: $1:\overline{2::2}:4$

$$2 \times 2 = \boxed{4}$$

Multiply the extremes: $1:2::2:4$

$$1 \times 4 = \boxed{4}$$

Determine if means = extremes.

$$4 = 4$$

By multiplying the means ($2 \times 2 = 4$) and multiplying the extremes ($1 \times 4 = 4$) we can see that the products are equal.

Solution: The proportion, $1:2::2:4$, is equal.

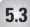

SKILL SHARPENER

Determine if the following proportions are equal.

1. $12:144::1:12$ _____

2. $24:250::48:600$ _____

3. $6:9::2:3$ _____

4. $100:10::1000:100$ _____

5. $230:10::23:1$ _____

6. $10:23::1:230$ _____

7. $234:43::23:4$ _____

8. $231:1::462:2$ _____

9. $231:1::243:2$ _____

10. $450:9000::1:20$ _____

Objective

5.4 Solve for a missing component in a proportion.

Often, one component of a proportion is unknown. Solve for the unknown component (x) as shown here.

The problem:

$$12 : x :: 6 : 1$$

Find the product of the means and the extremes.

    Multiply the means: $12 : x :: 6 : 1$

$$x \times 6 = 6x$$

Multiply the extremes: 12 : x :: 6 : 1

$$12 \times 1 = 12$$

Set up as:

$$6x = 12$$

To solve for x, divide each side by 6.

$$6x \div 6 = 1x \text{ (or just x)}$$

$$12 \div 6 = 2$$

$$x = 2$$

Solution: 12 : 2 :: 6 : 1

SKILL SHARPENER

Find the missing component (x) in each of the following proportions.

1. 12 : 6 :: x : 12   _____

2. 20 : x :: 1 : 10   _____

3. x : 34 :: 34 : 2   _____

4. 2.5 : 1 :: 10 : x   _____

5. 100 : 3 :: x : 900   _____

6. 4 : x :: 16 : 32   _____

7. x : 1 :: 11 : 1.5   _____

8. 50 : 3 :: 75 : x   _____

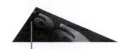

9. 67 : 100 :: 87 : x   _____

10. 78 : x :: 100 : 1   _____

Objective

5.5 Solve practical problems using proportions.

Proportions may be used to help solve many types of problems, including drug calculations. Consider the following examples.

Case # 1

You are asked to administer 65 milligrams of intravenous Lidocaine. You know that Lidocaine is packaged 100 mg. in a 5 milliliter prefilled syringe. How many milliliters of Lidocaine will you administer?

Set up your equation as follows by using the known factors. When using unlike terms like milligrams and milliliters, place like terms in places A and C and places B and D as illustrated here.

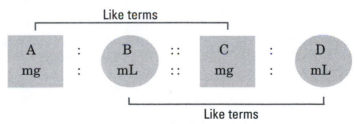

Set up as:

65 mg : x mL :: 100 mg : 5 mL

Find the product of the means and the extremes.

Multiply the means: 65 mg : x mL :: 100 mg : 5 mL

$100 \times x = 100x$

Multiply the extremes: 65 mg : x mL :: 100 mg : 5 mL

$65 \times 5 = 325$

Set up as:

$$100x = 325$$

To solve for x, divide each side by 100.

$$100x \div 100 = 1x \text{ or } x$$

$$325 \div 100 = 3.25$$

Solution: x = 3.25

Therefore, give 3.25 mL from the syringe to deliver 65 mg of Lidocaine.

Case # 2

Your gross pay is $1,800 and you paid $137.70 to FICA. What percentage of your gross pay is paid to FICA?

Since you know that $1,800 is 100% of your net pay, use 100 to compare against.

The problem:

$$137.70 : x :: 1,800 : 100$$

Find the product of the means and the extremes.

Multiply the means: $137.70 : x :: 1,800 : 100$

$$1,800 \times x = 1,800x$$

Multiply the extremes: $137.70 : x :: 1,800 : 100$

$$137.70 \times 100 = 13,770$$

Set up as:

$$1,800x = 13,770$$

To solve for x, divide each side by 1,800.

$$1,800x \div 1,800 = 1x \text{ or } x$$

$$13,770 \div 1,800 = 7.65$$

Solution: x = 7.65

Therefore, your FICA is 7.65% of your gross pay.

SKILL SHARPENER

Solve the following problems.

1. You are asked to administer 30 mg of a medication that is supplied in a 10 mL vial containing 100 mg. How many mL will you give to administer the ordered dose?

   _____

2. The physician orders 500 mg of amoxicillin for an adult patient. Amoxicillin is supplied in 125 mg tablets. How many tablets do you administer?

   _____

3. Acetaminophen is packaged in tablets of 325 mg. The physician asks you to give the resident 650 mg. How many tablets do you give?

   _____

4. You need to administer 4 mg of morphine sulfate (MS) slow IV push. MS is packaged 15 mg per mL. How many milliliters do you administer?

   _____

5. The ratio strength of a solution is 1:10. If there are 10 milliliters of the drug, how many milliliters of the solution are there?

   _____

6. While driving to work last week, you filled the tank of your new car with gasoline. The tank holds 16 gallons. You stopped today and topped off the tank by pumping 9.8 gallons. What percentage of the tank's capacity was left before you refilled the tank today?

   _____

7. Your hourly wage is $14. You are given the opportunity to work on Christmas Day at a rate of $2\frac{1}{2}$ times your normal hourly wage. How much will your hourly wage be if you work on Christmas Day?

_____

8. Your patient's urinary output for the shift was 120 mL. What percentage of her total urinary output (of 1,050 mL) for the day occurred on your shift?

_____

9. Your company contributes to your retirement fund based on a percentage of your income. You see that the company has contributed $150 to your retirement fund this month. What percentage of your $3,800 salary did your company contribute?

_____

10. You can purchase a gross (12 dozen) of 1-inch tape at 83 cents per roll. Individual rolls of the same tape are $1.02 each. Describe the amount (in percent) that you will save if you take advantage of buying tape in bulk.

_____

CONCLUSION

Knowing how to use ratios will help you to compare unlike items, and understanding how to solve for missing components in proportions will help you solve everyday problems encountered as a health care provider.

SELF-ASSESSMENT **POST-TEST**

Write the following ratios using colons. Reduce to lowest terms.

1. 7 patients out of 8 patients   _____

2. 3 ambulances out of 12 ambulances   _____

3. 33 surgeries out of 66 surgeries   _____

4. 9 prescriptions out of 27 prescriptions   _____

5. 20 days out of 30 days   _____

Determine if the following proportions are equal.

6. $124:10::1240:100$ _____

7. $90:15::4:2$ _____

8. $4:1::90:15$ _____

9. $75:19::5:1$ _____

10. $100:10::10:1$ _____

Solve for the missing component (x) in each of the following proportions.

11. $50:150::1:x$ _____

12. $180:x::12:24$ _____

13. $36:18::x:9$ _____

14. $x:900::300:1$ _____

15. $24:72::x:6$ _____

Solve the following problems using proportions.

16. You are asked to administer 75 milligrams (mg) of Lidocaine. It is packaged 10 mg per 1 milliliter (mL). How many mL do you administer?

_____

17. You have $1,238 of your total stock portfolio of $36,898 in international stocks. What percentage of your total stock portfolio is in international stocks?

_____

18. The physician asks you to administer 5 mg of atenolol to Mrs. Jones. Atenolol is packaged 1 mg per 2 mL. How many mL will you administer to Mrs. Jones?

_____

19. You are asked to administer 60 mg of furosemide to Mr. Genheim. The packaging you have on hand is 10 mg per mL in 4 mL ampules. How many ampules do you need?

_____

20. If 1/5 of the light bulbs in your house are 40 watts and lower, and there are 60 bulbs in your house, what percentage of bulbs in your house are 40 watts and lower?

_____

21. Your car gets 31 miles per gallon on the highway and 26 miles per gallon in the city. What percentage of mileage does your car get in the city compared to on the highway?

_____

22. You need to administer naloxone to Ms. Reed. The order is for 0.6 mg intramuscularly. Naloxone is packaged 0.4 mg/mL in 1 mL vials. How many mL do you administer?

_____

23. You have an adult patient that has second degree burns on approximately 2/3 of his anterior torso. Since you know that the entire anterior torso accounts for approximately 18% of total body surface area, determine what percentage of his total body surface area is burned.

---

24. Your teacher has developed a strange new grading system in which she requires that you attain at least 75% of the total points available to pass. You have obtained 1,132 points out of a possible 1,380. Did you pass the class?

---

25. Mrs. Reed's electrocardiogram reveals a QRS complex that is 30% wider than the normal limit of 0.12 seconds. How long is the QRS complex?

Percentages

LEARNING **OBJECTIVES**

After completing this chapter, the reader will be able to:

- **6.1** Define percent.
- **6.2** Convert decimals to percentages.
- **6.3** Convert percentages to decimals.
- **6.4** Solve to find a percent using multiplication and division.
- **6.5** Solve to find a percent using proportions.

KEY **TERM**

- percent

INTRODUCTION

Health care professionals use percentages in both their daily and professional lives for anything from figuring sale prices, sales tax, and tips to selecting appropriate intravenous solutions, medications, and assessing laboratory values (Figure 6-1). Percentages allow us to easily make comparisons and note changes based on a standard of 100.

Objective

 Define percent.

A **percent** is a part of one hundred. For example, 50% is 50 parts of 100. Though you could write this in other ways, using percentages sometimes makes it easier to understand. Health care providers utilize percentages for figuring discounts, strengths of solutions, and relative changes in anything from oxygen saturation to coronary artery blockage.

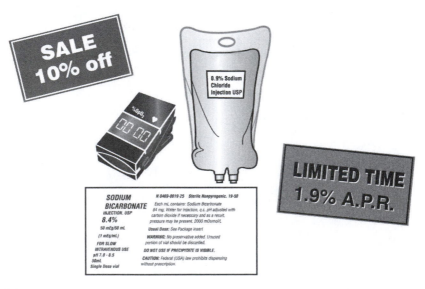

FIGURE 6-1 Whether you realize it or not, we use percentages on a daily basis.

Objective

6.2 Convert decimals to percentages.

To convert decimals to percentages, move the decimal two places to the right and add the % sign to the end. For example, 0.385 becomes 38.5% and 1.7625 becomes 176.25%.

SKILL SHARPENER

Convert the following decimals to percents.

1. 0.375 _____

2. 0.0932 _____

3. 1.832 _____

4. 0.9083 _____

5. 2.3323 _____

6. 0.3334 _____

7. 45.43243 _____

8. 1.232 _____

9. 0.9823 _____

10. 0.6676 _____

Objective

6.3 Convert percentages to decimals.

To convert percentages to decimals, remove the % sign and move the decimal two places to the left. For example, 59% would become 0.59.

Convert the following percentages to decimals.

1. 34% _____

2. 345% _____

3. 3.90% _____

4. 12.232% _____

5. 75.532% _____

6. 99.032% _____

7. 31.2594% _____

8. 54.433% _____

9. 8.45% _____

10. 92.322% _____

Objective

6.4 Solve to find a percent using multiplication and division.

To find a given percent of a number, convert the percentage to a decimal and multiply by the number.

The problem:

Find 63% of 94.

Convert percent to decimal.

63% = 0.63

Multiply.

$$0.63 \times 94$$

$$
\begin{array}{r}
94 \\
\times\ .63 \\
\hline
282 \\
564 \\
\hline
59.22
\end{array}
$$

Solution: 63% of 94 is 59.22

If using a calculator, use the % key.

The problem:

Find 24% of 75.

Push the following buttons to calculate:

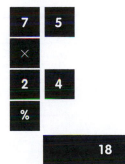

Solution:

    To find what percentage of one number another number is, simply divide the number that you want to find the percentage of into the other number. Convert the answer to a percentage.

The problem:

What % of 40 is 8?

Set up as:

$$8 \div 40 = \underline{}$$

Divide.

$$
\begin{array}{r}
.2 \\
40\overline{)8.0} \\
\underline{8\,0} \\
0\,0
\end{array}
$$

Convert to %.
$$0.2 \times 100 = 20\%$$
Solution: 8 is 20% of 40.

SKILL SHARPENER

Answer the following questions.

1. What is 75% of 350? _____

2. What is 40% of $12.95? _____

3. What is 99% of 250? _____

4. What is 12% of 32? _____

5. What is 25% of 3,200? _____

6. What is 19% of 15? _____

7. What is 5% of 150? _____

8. What is 34% of 88? _____

9. What is 65% of 65? _____

10. What is 8% of 185? _____

11. What percentage of 12 is 4? _____

12. What percentage of 900 is 180? _____

13. What percentage of 750 is 50? _____

14. What percentage of 120 is 100? _____

15. What percentage of 300 is 75? _____

16. What percentage of 250 is 75?   _____

17. What percentage of 76 is 14?   _____

18. What percentage of 88 is 3?   _____

19. What percentage of 12.5 is 8?   _____

20. What percentage of 3.5 is 1.25?   _____

Objective

6.5 Solve to find a percent using proportions.

Another way to find a percent is by using proportions. Set up your proportion by using **x** to indicate the unknown factor and **100** to signify 100%.

The problem:

What % of 150 is 120?

Note: Since we are finding a percentage (part of 100) we will use 100 as the whole.

Because 150 is the other whole, set up the equation as:

x : 100 :: 120 : 150

Multiply the means: x : 100 :: 120 : 150

$100 \times 120 = 12{,}000$

Multiply the extremes: x : 100 :: 120 : 150

$150 \times x = 150x$

Set up as:

$12{,}000 = 150x$

To solve for x, divide each side by 150.

$12{,}000 \div 150 = 80$

$150x \div 150 = 1x \text{ or } x$

Solution: x = 80

Therefore, 80 : 100 :: 120 : 150 or 120 is 80% of 150.

By utilizing proportions, you can determine the missing component regardless which component is missing.

SKILL SHARPENER

Solve the following word problems using proportions.

1. What is 34% of 325? _____

2. What is 75% of 150? _____

3. What is 12.5% of 325? _____

4. What is 34.58% of 76? _____

5. What is 1.9% of 768? _____

6. What is 5.47% of 9,380? _____

7. What is 3.75% of 36? _____

8. What is 7% of 99? _____

9. What is 33.35% of 190? _____

10. What is 5.8% of 346? _____

11. What percentage of 150 is 18.75? _____

12. What percentage of 398 is 294.52? _____

13. What percentage of 125 is 27.5? _____

14. What percentage of 1,395 is 153.45? _____

15. What percentage of 69 is 35.88? _____

16. What percentage of 12 is 4.32? _____

17. What percentage of 1,965 is 137.55? _____

18. What percentage of 550 is 247.5? _____

19. What percentage of 475 is 460.75? _____

20. What percentage of 1,200 is 30.72? _____

CONCLUSION

Percentages are used in many ways, in both health care and daily life, to make numbers and relationships between numbers easier to understand. The ability to convert from decimals to percentages and percentages to decimals, along with the ability to find a percentage using multiplication, division, and proportions, will be beneficial in both your professional career and your personal life.

SELF-ASSESSMENT **POST-TEST**

Convert the following decimals to percentages.

1. 0.45 _____

2. 0.78 _____

3. 0.89 _____

4. 0.91 _____

5. 0.3341 _____

6. 0.2556 _____

7. 0.873 _____

8. 0.112 _____

9. 0.494 _____

10. 1.00 _____

Convert the following percentages to decimals.

11. 34% _____

12. 57% _____

13. 12% _____

14. 90% _____

15. 43% _____

16. 75.67% _____

17. 39.44% _____

18. 11.901% _____

19. 85.554% _____

20. 22.450% _____

Answer the following percentage problems.

21. What is 75% of 350? _____

22. What is 25.5% of 79? _____

23. What is 99% of 1,200? _____

24. What is 23.98% of 125? _____

25. What is 78.9% of 13,323? _____

26. What is 1.2% of 5? _____

27. What is 9.9% of 34? _____

28. What is 14.95% of 78,000? _____

29. What is 67% of 32? _____

30. What is 30% of 9? _____

31. 35.1 is what percentage of 78? _____

32. 9.75 is what percentage of 39? _____

33. 111.28 is what percentage of 856? _____

34. 705 is what percentage of 965.8? _____

35. 5.32 is what percentage of 38? _____

36. 56 is what percentage of 175? _____

37. 0.45 is what percentage of 15? _____

38. 47.4 is what percentage of 395? _____

39. 4.5 is what percentage of 250? _____

40. 124.56 is what percentage of 1,384? _____

41. You purchase a television set for $599 and must pay the 9% sales tax. What is your total cost?

_____

42. You receive a 7% discount on a purchase of $1,275. What is your discounted cost?

_____

43. Your patient's pulse rate is 30% higher than its normal rate of 80. What is her pulse rate?

_____

44. All the supplies in the emergency clinic are charged at cost plus 20%. What price would you charge for an item costing $14.75?

_____

45. The local fitness club offers memberships for $40 per month. Hospital employees are eligible for a 25% discount. What is the discounted monthly rate for hospital employees?

_____

46. Your patient's IV bag holds 1000 mL of normal saline. You see that 350 mL is left. What percentage of the saline has been infused?

_____

47. A baseball player reaches base 186 times in 350 at bats. What percentage of the time does he reach base? Round to the nearest hundredth.

_____

48. Your passbook savings account pays 3.75% interest on your $3,575 balance. How much interest have you earned?

_____

49. How much sales tax would you pay on a purchase of $3.50 based upon a sales tax rate of 8.75%?

_____

50. Your hospital reports that 555 of the hospital's 1,500 employees will be eligible for retirement next year. What percentage of the hospital's employees will be eligible for retirement?

_____

Conversions

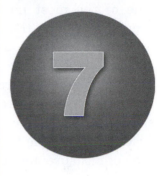

LEARNING **OBJECTIVES**

After completing this chapter, the reader will be able to:

- **7.1** Convert from decimal to fraction.
- **7.2** Convert from decimal to percent.
- **7.3** Convert from fraction to decimal.
- **7.4** Convert from fraction to percent.
- **7.5** Convert from percent to fraction.
- **7.6** Convert from percent to decimal.
- **7.7** Convert units of measure within the metric system.
- **7.8** Convert units of measure within the apothecary system.
- **7.9** Convert units of measure within the household system.
- **7.10** Convert between the apothecary, household, and metric systems.

KEY **TERM**

- conversion

INTRODUCTION

One of the most important mathematical skills health care providers need is the ability to convert from one unit of measurement to another. **Conversion** is the act of changing from one system or measurement to another. Sometimes this skill involves conversion from a decimal to a percent. Sometimes it involves conversions to or from fractions. It may involve conversion between measurement systems. This chapter helps you practice converting from one type of number to another and one type of measurement system to another.

Objective

7.1 Convert from decimal to fraction.

Sometimes you will need to convert from a decimal to a fraction. To do this, follow the steps outlined below.

The problem:

Convert 0.84 to a fraction.

Since we know that 0.84 is equal to $\frac{84}{100}$, we can convert to $\frac{84}{100}$ and reduce.

To reduce, find the greatest common factor (GCF) of the numerator and denominator.

84	**100**
$1 \times 84 = 84$	$1 \times 100 = 100$
$2 \times 42 = 84$	$2 \times 50 = 100$
$4 \times 21 = 84$	$4 \times 25 = 100$

The GCF is 4.

Divide the numerator and denominator by the GCF.

$$\frac{84}{100} \div \frac{4}{4} = \frac{21}{25}$$

Solution: $0.84 = \frac{21}{25}$

SKILL SHARPENER

Convert the following decimals to fractions. Reduce to lowest terms.

1. 0.38   _____

2. 0.97   _____

3. 0.233   _____

4. 0.125   _____

5. 0.25   _____

6. 0.75   _____

7. 0.9   _____

8. 1.23   _____

9. 2.75   _____

10. 3.5   _____

Objective

7.2 Convert from decimal to percent.

To convert from a decimal to a percent, move the decimal two places to the right and add a % sign. For example, 0.50 equals 50%.

Convert the following decimals to percents.

1. 0.34 _____

2. 0.25 _____

3. 0.87 _____

4. 0.67 _____

5. 0.39 _____

6. 0.2 _____

7. 0.9 _____

8. 0.123 _____

9. 1.23 _____

10. 2.78 _____

Objective

7.3 Convert from fraction to decimal.

To convert a fraction to a decimal, divide the denominator into the numerator. The quotient is your answer.

The problem:

Convert $\frac{3}{5}$ to a decimal.

Set up as:

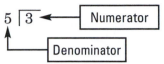

Divide.

$$
\begin{array}{r}
0.6 \\
5\overline{\smash{)}3.0} \\
\underline{3\,0} \\
0
\end{array}
$$

Solution: $\frac{3}{5} = 0.6$

If the dividend repeats the same digit, place a line over the repeating digits or use rounding to complete your answer. Consider this example.

The problem:

Convert $\frac{1}{3}$ to a decimal.

Set up as:

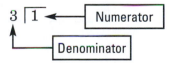

Divide.

$$
\begin{array}{r}
0.333 \\
3\overline{\smash{)}1.000} \\
\underline{9} \\
10 \\
\underline{9} \\
10
\end{array}
$$

Solution: $\frac{1}{3} = 0.\overline{33}$

Since the 3 will keep repeating indefinitely, place a line over the 3s.

Convert the following fractions to decimals.

1. $\frac{1}{2}$ _____

2. $\frac{2}{3}$ _____

3. $\frac{4}{5}$ _____

4. $\frac{7}{16}$ _____

5. $\frac{9}{10}$ _____

6. $\frac{32}{100}$ _____

7. $\frac{3}{8}$ _____

8. $\frac{8}{16}$ _____

9. $\frac{3}{9}$ _____

10. $\frac{125}{1000}$ _____

Objective

 7.4 Convert from fraction to percent.

To convert from a fraction to a percent, first convert the fraction to a decimal. To accomplish this, divide the denominator into the numerator.

The problem:

Convert $\frac{3}{8}$ to a percent.

Set up as:

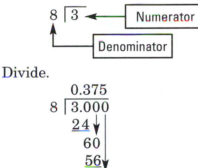

Divide.

$$
\begin{array}{r}
0.375 \\
8\,\overline{\smash{)}\,3.000} \\
\underline{24} \\
60 \\
\underline{56} \\
40
\end{array}
$$

Convert decimal to percent by moving the decimal two spaces to the right and add the % sign.

0.37.5

Solution: $\frac{3}{8} = 37.5\%$

SKILL SHARPENER

Convert the following fractions to percents.

1. $\frac{4}{5}$ _____

2. $\frac{2}{3}$ _____

3. $\frac{1}{8}$ _____

4. $\frac{6}{7}$ _____

5. $\frac{3}{9}$ _____

6. $\frac{12}{36}$ _____

7. $\frac{23}{45}$ _____

8. $\frac{45}{150}$ _____

9. $\frac{7}{16}$ _____

10. $\frac{8}{32}$ _____

Objective

7.5 Convert from percent to fraction.

To convert from a percent to a fraction, first convert the percent to a decimal. That decimal number should be used as the numerator and the denominator should be 100. Then reduce to the lowest terms.

The problem:

Convert 37% to a fraction.

Convert to a decimal by dropping the % sign and moving the decimal two places to the left.

37%

0.37. | Drop % and move decimal two places to the left.

0.37

Since we know that 0.37 is equal to $\frac{37}{100}$, we should now reduce to lowest terms.

To reduce, find the GCF of the numerator and denominator.

37	100
1 × 37 = 37	1 × 100 = 100
	2 × 50 = 100
	4 × 25 = 100
	5 × 20 = 100
	10 × 10 = 100

Since the GCF is 1, this cannot be reduced any further.

Solution: 37% = $\frac{37}{100}$

Convert the following percents to fractions. Reduce to lowest terms.

1. 23% _____

2. 45% _____

3. 90% _____

4. 50% _____

5. 33% _____

6. 65% _____

7. 60% _____

8. 12% _____

9. 9% _____

10. 125% _____

Objective

7.6 Convert from percent to decimal.

When converting from a percent to a decimal, simply drop the % sign and move the decimal two places to the left.

The problem:

Convert 98% to a decimal.

Drop the % sign and move the decimal two places to the left.

> 98%
>
> 0.98.
>
> 0.98

Solution: 98% = 0.98

SKILL SHARPENER

Convert the following percents to decimals.

1. 32% _____

2. 15% _____

3. 67% _____

4. 324% _____

5. 3% _____

6. 13%   _____

7. 91%   _____

8. 0.38%   _____

9. 0.9%   _____

10. 12%   _____

Objective

7.7 Convert units of measure within the metric system.

Since the metric system is based on units of ten, conversion requires that you multiply or divide. This is made especially simple since multiplication and division may be accomplished by moving decimals to the right or left.

To multiply by 10, move the decimal one place to the right.

Example

$39.84 \times 10 =$

39.84

398.4

To multiply by 100   —   move the decimal 2 places to the right.

To multiply by 1,000   —   move the decimal 3 places to the right.

To multiply by 10,000 — move the decimal 4 places to the right.

To multiply by 100,000 — move the decimal 5 places to the right.

To divide by 10, move the decimal one place to the left.

Example

39.84 ÷ 10 =

39.84

3.984

To divide by 100 — move the decimal 2 places to the left.

To divide by 1,000 — move the decimal 3 places to the left.

To divide by 10,000 — move the decimal 4 places to the left.

To divide by 100,000 — move the decimal 5 places to the left.

SKILL SHARPENER

Convert the following measurements.

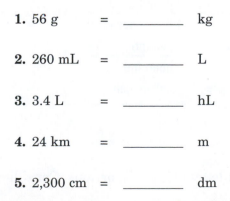

1. 56 g = _____ kg

2. 260 mL = _____ L

3. 3.4 L = _____ hL

4. 24 km = _____ m

5. 2,300 cm = _____ dm

6. 0.5 L   = _____ mL

7. 29 mg   = _____ g

8. 3,400 mg = _____ g

9. 2.3 L   = _____ mL

10. 0.125 L   = _____ mL

Objective

7.8 Convert units of measure within the apothecary system.

To convert units of measure within the apothecary system, refer to the conversion chart shown in Figure 7-1.

60 grains (gr)	=	1 dram (dr) ʒ
8 drams (dr)	=	1 ounce (oz) ℥
12 ounces (oz)	=	1 pound (lb)
60 minims (♏)	=	1 fluidram (fldr)
8 fluidrams (fldr)	=	1 fluidounce (floz)
16 fluidounces (floz)	=	1 pint (pt)
2 pints (pt)	=	1 quart (qt)
4 quarts (qt)	=	1 gallon (gal)

FIGURE 7-1 Apothecary equivalents

Conversions may easily be made by using proportions. Consider the following example.

The problem:

> The medication order reads ℥ss. You need to figure how many grains to administer.

Since we know that 1 dram is equivalent to 60 grains, set up the problem as a proportion.

Set up as:

$$\frac{1}{2} \text{ dram} : x \text{ grains} :: 1 \text{ dram} : 60 \text{ grains}$$

Multiply the means. $\frac{1}{2} : x :: 1 : 60$

$$1 \times x = 1x \text{ or } x$$

Multiply the extremes. $\frac{1}{2} : x :: 1 : 60$

$$\frac{1}{2} \times 60 = 30$$

Solution: x = 30

Therefore, $\frac{1}{2}$ dram = 30 grains.

SKILL SHARPENER

Convert the following measurements.

1. 60 gr = _____ dr

2. 2 dr = _____ gr

3. 16 floz = _____ pt

4. 2 pt = _____ qt

5. 4 fldr = _____ ℳ

6. 8 fldr = _____ floz

7. 2 gal = _____ qt

8. 1 gal = _____ pt

9. 480 ℳ = _____ floz

10. 1 fldr = _____ ℠

Objective

7.9 Convert units of measure within the household system.

To convert units of measure within the household system, refer to the conversion chart in Figure 7-2.

60 gtt	=	1 t or tsp		
3 t or tsp	=	1 T		
180 gtt	=	1 T	=	$\frac{1}{2}$ oz
2 T	=	1 oz	=	6 t or tsp
360 gtt	=	2 T		
1 oz	=	30 cc or 30 mL		
6 oz	=	1 tcp		
8 oz	=	1 C or 1 glass		
2 C	=	1 pt	=	16 oz
2 pt	=	1 qt	=	32 oz
4 C	=	1 qt	=	32 oz
4 qt	=	1 gal	=	128 oz

FIGURE 7-2 Household equivalents

Make conversions using proportions as illustrated here.

The problem:

> Your patient needs 30 mL of a liquid medication. You know that 30 mL is equivalent to 1 ounce, and $\frac{1}{2}$ ounce is roughly equivalent to 1 T.

Set up as:

30 mL : x T :: 15 mL : 1 T

Multiply the means.　30 : x :: 15 : 1

x × 15 = 15x

Multiply the extremes.　30 : x :: 15 : 1

30 × 1 = 30

Set up as:

15x = 30

To solve for x, divide both sides by 15.

15x ÷ 15 = 1x or x

30 ÷ 15 = 2

Solution: x = 2

Therefore, 2 T = 30 mL.

SKILL SHARPENER

Convert the following measurements.

1. 60 drops　　=　　_____　t

2. 240 drops   =   _____   T

3. 1 glass   =   _____   ounces

4. 1 cup   =   _____   oz

5. 1 oz   =   _____   T

6. 1 T   =   _____   t

7. 4 T   =   _____   oz

8. 1 ounce   =   _____   drops

9. 12 ounces   =   _____   cup

10. 3 T   =   _____   t

Objective

7.10 Convert between the apothecary, household, and metric systems.

Health care providers are frequently asked to convert from one measurement system to another. It is important that care is taken to assure accuracy in conversions. Since proportions may be used to compare unlike items, it is an ideal method to convert between the systems of measurement. Appendix C contains conversion charts for the three common systems of measurement.

The problem:

> You need to instruct a patient how to take 8 drams (℥) of a medication. Since you know that one dram is equivalent to 2 teaspoons, convert to a measure that the patient can use at home.

Set up as:

8 drams : x tsp :: 1 dram : 2 tsp

Multiply the means.   8 : x :: 1 : 2

x × 1 = 1x or x

Multiply the extremes.   8 : x :: 1 : 2

8 × 2 = 16

Solution: x = 16

Therefore, to take 8 drams, the patient must take 16 tsp.

What is another way you could make it easier for the patient to take the medicine? Could you convert to another household measure?

Convert the following measurements using proportions.

1. 1 oz   = _____   gtts

2. 1 pt   = _____   mL

3. 60 mL   = _____   drop

4. 1 T   = _____   gtts

5. 1 T   = _____   mL

6. 4 T   = _____   mL

7. 30 ℳ   = _____   mL

8. 2 floz   = _____   mL

9. 10 mL   = _____   fl ℥

10. 1 floz = _____   T

CONCLUSION

Using the skills in this chapter, you should be able to make necessary conversions between fractions, decimals, and percents. Though it may not be necessary to perform these conversions on a daily basis, the ability to perform these conversions will make your job as a health care professional easier and will help you to provide the best care for your patients.

Your ability to convert between each of the three systems of measurement is important in assuring that patients receive the correct dosages of medications, both while in your care and at home. It is helpful to memorize some of the common conversions and to keep a chart, like the one in Appendix C, handy for those less common conversions.

SELF-ASSESSMENT **POST-TEST**

Convert the following to fractions.

1. 0.44 _____

2. 0.68 _____

3. 0.23 _____

4. 0.11 _____

5. 0.98 _____

Convert the following to percents.

6. 0.46 _____

7. 0.125 _____

8. 0.33 _____

9. 0.87 _____

10. 0.58 _____

Convert the following to decimals.

11. $\frac{4}{9}$ _____

12. $\frac{9}{10}$ _____

13. $\frac{34}{50}$ _____

14. $\frac{22}{40}$ _____

15. $\frac{12}{15}$ _____

Convert the following to percents.

16. $\frac{41}{55}$ _____

17. $\frac{3}{8}$ _____

18. $\frac{6}{90}$ _____

19. $\frac{2}{3}$ _____

20. $\frac{4}{11}$ _____

Convert the following to fractions.

21. 34% _____

22. 57% _____

23. 87% _____

24. 66% _____

25. 12% _____

Convert the following to decimals.

26. 13% _____

27. 61% _____

28. 59% _____

29. 31% _____

30. 98% _____

150

Convert the following measurements.

31. 3 g = _____ kg

32. 12 km = _____ m

33. 1300 mg = _____ g

34. 0.595 l = _____ mL

35. 4 dr = _____ gr

36. 16 fl ʒ = _____ fl ʒ

37. 4 pt = _____ qt

38. 540 drops = _____ T

39. 2 glasses = _____ fluidounces

40. 4 T = _____ t

This unit allows the student to apply the skills learned in Unit One to actual examples that are relevant and mimic those experienced in the work place. Through practice, these operations will become second nature as they develop into part of the health care professional's daily routine.

Though some operations may seem routine, students should realize that accuracy is imperative, and attention to detail is crucial in assuring that patients receive the best possible care.

Medication Dosage Calculations

LEARNING **OBJECTIVES**

After completing this chapter, the reader will be able to:

8.1 List the components of a typical medication label.

8.2 Read a medication label.

8.3 Read a prescription.

8.4 Read a syringe.

8.5 Determine the amount of fluid remaining in an intravenous bag.

8.6 Calculate intravenous drip rates.

8.7 Determine the concentration of solutions.

8.8 Calculate medication dosages using proportions.

8.9 Convert medication dosages for home use.

KEY **TERMS**

- concentration of a solution
- drip rate
- expiration date
- generic name
- KVO line
- lot number
- macrodrip
- medication label
- microdrip
- percent strength
- piggyback
- prescription
- syringe
- TKO line
- trade name

INTRODUCTION

Health care providers deal with medication dosages and solution strengths in a number of ways. Your ability to perform mathematical calculations and accurately read medication orders and labels will help assure that patients receive the correct dosages and strengths of the intended medicines. Additionally, it is important that you be able to interpret medication orders and convert medication orders to household measurements so that patients accurately measure their medications using household devices.

Objective

8.1 List the components of a typical medication label.

It is important that health care professionals be able to read a **medication label**. These labels contain important information that helps the health care professional to assure that the right medication at the right strength is delivered to the patient. Though the style of medication labels varies, certain components should be common to each label.

NDC 0002-5058-18
75 mL (When Mixed) M-5058

℞ Lilly

CECLOR®
(CEFACLOR) FOR
ORAL SUSPENSION
USP
250 mg
per 5 mL

CAUTION—Federal (USA) law
prohibits dispensing without
prescription.

0002-5058-18   PULL

N 3   6

Usual Dose—Pediatric patients, 20 mg per kg a day (40 mg per kg in otitis media) in three divided doses. Adults, 250 mg three times a day. See literature for complete dosage information.
Contains Cefaclor Monohydrate equivalent to 3.75 g anhydrous Cefaclor in a dry pleasantly flavored mixture.
Prior to Mixing, Store at Controlled Room Temperature 59° to 86°F (15° to 30°C)
Directions for Mixing—Add 45 mL of water in two portions to the dry mixture in the bottle. Shake well after each addition.
Each 5 mL (Approx. one teaspoonful) will then contain: Cefaclor Monohydrate equivalent to 250 mg anhydrous Cefaclor.

Eli Lilly and Company
Indianapolis, IN 46285, USA

Expiration Date

WV 6475 AMX

75 mL CECLOR® CEFACLOR FOR ORAL SUSPENSION, USP
250 mg per 5 mL. Oversize bottle provides extra space for shaking. Store in a refrigerator. May be kept for 14 days without significant loss of potency. Keep Tightly Closed. Discard unused portion after 14 days. SHAKE WELL BEFORE USING

Control No.

Trade name – Also referred to as brand name of the medication

Generic name – The nonproprietary name of the medication

Manufacturer – The company that manufactured the medication

National Drug Code (NDC) number – A number used to identify the manufacturer, the medication, and the container size

Dosage strength – Amount of medication contained within a given dose (in this example, 250 mg per 5 mL)

Drug form – Whether a liquid, capsule, drop, tablet, and so on

Usual adult dose – The typical adult dose for the common use of the medicine

Total amount enclosed – Number of tablets, approximate number of drops, ounces, or milliliters

Prescription warning – Denotes that this medication is available by prescription only

Expiration date – Denotes the last date in which this medication should be used (Since this label is for purposes of illustration, no expiration date is visible.)

Lot or control number – The lot number would be applied before shipping the actual product (In this example, there is no lot number visible.)

Find the requested information on each of the following medication labels or boxes. If you are unable to see one of the requested items, write "NOT SEEN" on the line.

1.

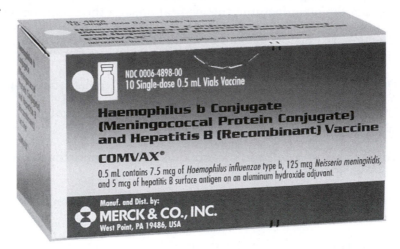

NDC 0006-4898-00
10 Single-dose 0.5 mL Vials Vaccine

**Haemophilus b Conjugate
(Meningococcal Protein Conjugate)
and Hepatitis B (Recombinant) Vaccine**

COMVAX®

0.5 mL contains 7.5 mcg of *Haemophilus influenzae* type b, 125 mcg *Neisseria meningitidis*, and 5 mcg of hepatitis B surface antigen on an aluminum hydroxide adjuvant.

Manuf. and Dist. by:
MERCK & CO., INC.
West Point, PA 19486, USA

Trade name	_____
Generic name	_____
Manufacturer	_____
NDC number	_____
Dosage strength	_____
Drug form	_____
Usual adult dose	_____
Amount enclosed	_____
Prescription warning	_____
Expiration date	_____
Lot number	_____

2.

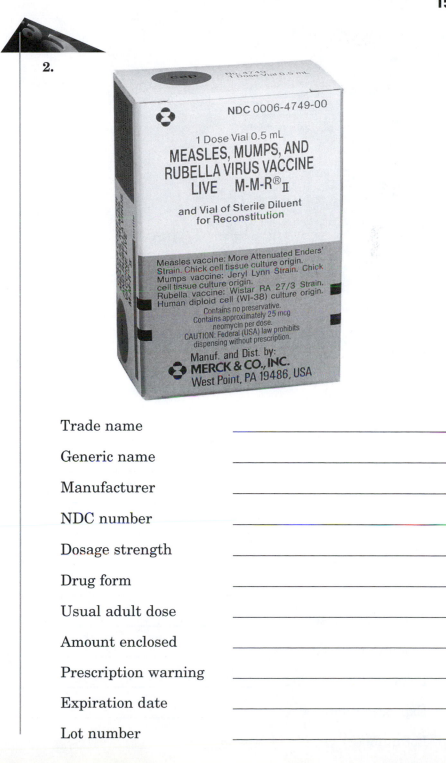

NDC 0006-4749-00

1 Dose Vial 0.5 mL
MEASLES, MUMPS, AND
RUBELLA VIRUS VACCINE
LIVE   M-M-R® II

and Vial of Sterile Diluent
for Reconstitution

Measles vaccine: More Attenuated Enders'
Strain. Chick cell tissue culture origin.
Mumps vaccine: Jeryl Lynn Strain. Chick
cell tissue culture origin.
Rubella vaccine: Wistar RA 27/3 Strain.
Human diploid cell (WI-38) culture origin.
Contains no preservative.
Contains approximately 25 mcg
neomycin per dose.
CAUTION: Federal (USA) law prohibits
dispensing without prescription.
Manuf. and Dist. by:
MERCK & CO., INC.
West Point, PA 19486, USA

Trade name	_____
Generic name	_____
Manufacturer	_____
NDC number	_____
Dosage strength	_____
Drug form	_____
Usual adult dose	_____
Amount enclosed	_____
Prescription warning	_____
Expiration date	_____
Lot number	_____

3.

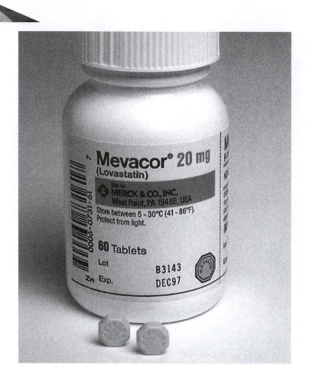

Trade name   _____

Generic name   _____

Manufacturer   _____

NDC number   _____

Dosage strength   _____

Drug form   _____

Usual adult dose   _____

Amount enclosed   _____

Prescription warning   _____

Expiration date   _____

Lot number   _____

4.

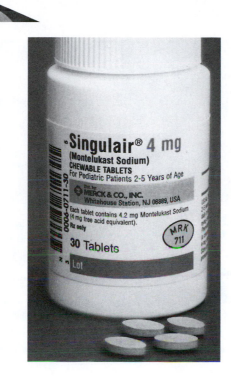

Trade name

Generic name

Manufacturer

NDC number

Dosage strength

Drug form

Usual adult dose

Amount enclosed

Prescription warning

Expiration date

Lot number

5.

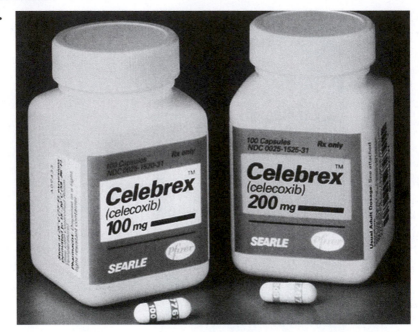

Trade name _____

Generic name _____

Manufacturer _____

NDC number _____

Dosage strength _____

Drug form _____

Usual adult dose _____

Amount enclosed _____

Prescription warning _____

Expiration date _____

Lot number _____

Objective

8.2 Read a medication label.

By understanding the components of a medication label, you can then read a medication label with understanding. From this label, you should be able to differentiate between the trade name and the generic name. The **trade name** is typically shown more prominently than the generic name and usually carries a ® or ™ symbol to denote a registered trademark. The **generic name** is a nonproprietary name that is used to designate a medication that is not protected by trademark.

The manufacturer's name should be apparent, as should be the NDC number. The dosage strength should be easily found and is sometimes incorporated into the trade name. Other items like the dosage strength, form, normal adult dose, and total amount enclosed should also be quite apparent. The prescription warning, which reads *CAUTION: Federal (USA) law prohibits dispensing without a prescription*, should be located on each label for prescription medications.

The **expiration date** denotes the last date in which the medication should be used. The **lot number** is an internal reference number used by the manufacturer so that medications may be traced to the day and the batch in which they were manufactured. Lot numbers are used for tracking and quality control and are vitally important should a recall occur.

From the information contained on each medication label, answer the following questions.

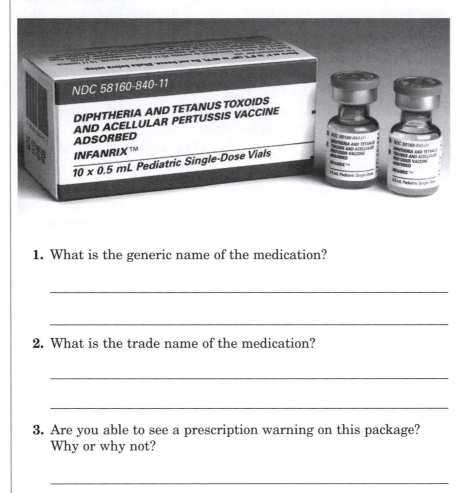

NDC 58160-840-11

DIPHTHERIA AND TETANUS TOXOIDS AND ACELLULAR PERTUSSIS VACCINE ADSORBED

INFANRIX™

10 x 0.5 mL Pediatric Single-Dose Vials

1. What is the generic name of the medication?

_____

_____

2. What is the trade name of the medication?

_____

_____

3. Are you able to see a prescription warning on this package? Why or why not?

_____

_____

4. What is the typical dose of this medication?

_____

_____

5. What is the dosage strength?

_____

_____

6. What is the total volume contained in this package?

_____

_____

7. Who is the manufacturer of this medication?

_____

_____

8. What is the NDC number?

_____

_____

9. What other components of the label should you look for?

_____

_____

10. What other information can you garner from reading this label?

_____

_____

Objective

8.3 Read a prescription.

In the same way that physicians write medication orders for patients in health care facilities, they also write prescriptions so that their patients are able to purchase medication for home use. A **prescription** is a medication order that a physician writes or telephones to the patient's local pharmacy. Like the medication label, the information must contain certain components that are common to all prescriptions (Figure 8-1). These components include:

- Physician's name, address, telephone number, and registration number

- The patient's name and address

- The date the prescription is written

- The superscription, $R_{\not\!\!/}$, which means take thou

- The inscription that states the name of the medication

- The subscription that gives directions for filling the prescription

- The signature, designated by the abbreviation Sig, provides directions to the patient for taking the medication

- Signature lines for the physician to sign indicating if a generic substitute is allowed or if the prescription must be dispensed as written

- Refill blank where the physician indicates the number of times the prescription may be refilled (by circling a number) or if no refills are allowed (designated by NR)

- A designation to the pharmacist to label the medication properly

Lane Kennamer, MD
1212 Liberty Parkway • Birmingham, AL 35023
(205) 555-1438

Date _____

Name _____

Address _____

℞

Generic Substitution Allowed _____
                                                                    M.D.

Dispense As Written _____
                                                                    M.D.

REPETATUR NR 1 2 3 p.r.n.   Reg# _____

[ ] LABEL

FIGURE 8-1 Sample prescription

Using the prescription shown, answer the following questions.

Lane Kennamer, MD

1212 Liberty Parkway • Birmingham, AL 35023

(205) 555-1438

Date _____

Name _Dora Reid_____

Address _____

R⅄ _Tussionex susp. #240 ml_

Sig 1 tsp po ℞ 12 hr.

Generic Substitution Allowed _Lane Kennamer_____
M.D.

Dispense As Written _____
M.D.

REPETATUR NR 1 ②3 p.r.n. Reg# _____

☑ LABEL

---

1. Who is the prescribing physician?

_____

2. What is his/her office telephone number?

_____

3. Who is the patient?

_____

4. What medication is prescribed?

_____

5. What is the dosage strength of the medication?

_____

6. How much will be dispensed?

_____

7. Are refills prescribed?

_____

8. Can the pharmacist offer a generic equivalent (if available)?

_____

9. What does the symbol ℞ mean?

_____

10. Using this mock prescription, write a concise set of instructions explaining how to take this medication, how often, and so on. Use the abbreviation list in Appendix B if necessary.

_____

_____

Objective

8.4 Read a syringe.

Syringes are used to administer precise amounts of medication, either through injections into the skin or muscle or through infusions into an intravenous line. Marked with a series of graduations to indicate volume, syringes come in a variety of sizes, but are read in the same manner. The syringe should be read at the edge of the plunger nearest the needle. This point indicates the remaining volume of solution in the syringe.

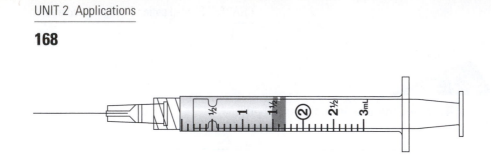

In this example, there is 1 1/2 mL remaining in the syringe. Assuming the syringe started with 3 mL, 1 1/2 mL has been administered.

SKILL SHARPENER

Determine the amount of solution remaining in each of the following syringes.

1. _____

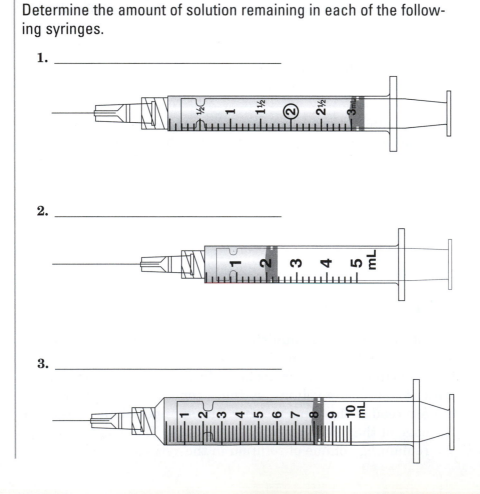

2. _____

3. _____

4. _____

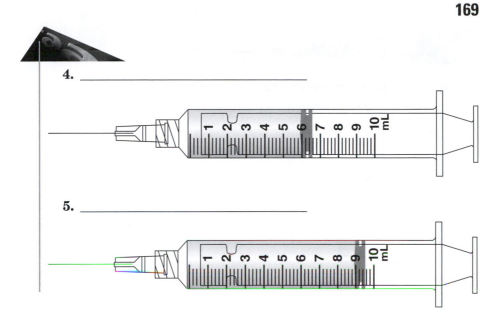

5. _____

Objective

8.5 Determine the amount of fluid remaining in an intravenous bag.

Intravenous fluids come in both glass bottles and plastic bags. To measure the amount of fluid infused, note the level of the fluid. The marking that is even with the top of the fluid solution will tell you the amount of fluid remaining. To determine how much fluid has been infused, subtract the fluid remaining from the capacity of the bag.

IV bags are commonly supplied as 250 mL, 500 mL, or 1,000 mL. Smaller bags of 100 mL are available to mix certain medications. Check the capacity of the IV bag by noting the capacity displayed on the bag.

The bag illustrated here is a 1,000 mL bag. Also, note that the current level is at 2, indicating that 200 mL of fluid has been infused and 800 mL remains.

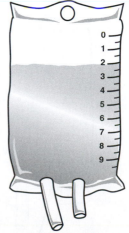

1,000 mL − 200 mL = 800 mL

Indicate both the volume remaining and the amount infused in each of the following examples.

1. Volume remaining:

_____

Amount infused:

_____

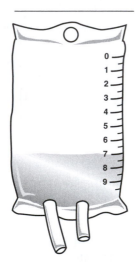

2. Volume remaining:

_____

Amount infused:

_____

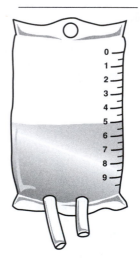

3. Volume remaining:

_____

Amount infused:

_____

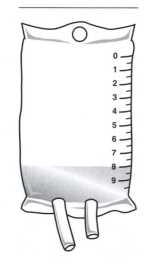

4. Volume remaining:

_____

Amount infused:

_____

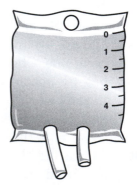

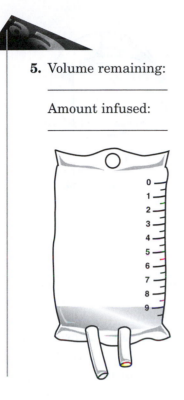

5. Volume remaining:

_____

Amount infused:

_____

Objective

8.6 Calculate intravenous drip rates.

The rate of intravenous fluid infusions is controlled by either gravity-fed hand controls or electronic pumps. Electronic pumps require only that you set the desired rate of infusion. When controlling infusions that are not on a pump, a mathematical formula is used to calculate **drip rates**, or the rate in which the fluid drips from the IV bag into the intravenous line.

Two common types of drip sets exist. Sometimes called standard sets, **macrodrip** sets are commonly used for fluid replacement and to keep a route available for intravenous medications (Figure 8-2). Intravenous lines, started for the sole purpose of assuring intravenous access, are sometimes referred to as **TKO lines** or **KVO lines** because they are run at a rate sufficient only "to keep open" or to "keep vein open." Macrodrip sets

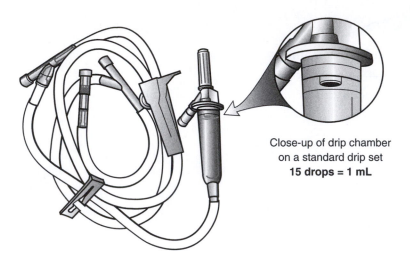

FIGURE 8-2 A macrodrip set is sometimes referred to as a standard set.

are typically available as 10-, 12-, or 15-drop sets. These numbers refer to how many drops it takes to equal one mL of fluid. In other words, a 15-drop set delivers one mL for every 15 drops of fluid that drips through the set.

A **microdrip** set is utilized when there is a need to limit the volume of fluid infused (Figure 8-3). Microdrip sets deliver

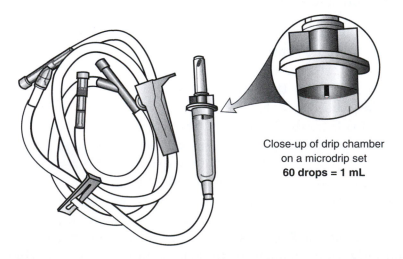

FIGURE 8-3 A microdrip set is sometimes referred to as a minidrip set.

one mL for every 60 (smaller) drops of fluid that drips through the set.

The following formula is used to determine how to adjust the drip set to administer the desired amount of fluid over the prescribed time.

amount to be infused × drip set ÷ time of infusion (in minutes) = number of drops per minute to be infused

Example

You are asked to infuse 250 mL over 3 hours. Your hospital uses a 15-drop-per-mL drip set.

amount × drip set ÷ time (in minutes) = drops per minute to be infused

$$250 \times 15 = 3{,}750$$

$$3{,}750 \div 180 = 20.8\overline{33}$$

Therefore, you will need to adjust the IV to drip approximately once every three seconds to deliver 250 mL in three hours.

When a constant infusion of medication is given over time, **piggyback** infusions may be used. A piggyback is a secondary infusion that is attached to an already existing (primary) IV line. The primary line is turned off and the piggybacked line delivers the necessary infusion of medication.

SKILL SHARPENER

Figure the drip rate for the following scenarios.

1. You are asked to administer 1,000 mL of normal saline over 24 hours using a 15-drop-per-mL set.

_____

2. You need to adjust the flow rate of an existing IV line to administer 200 mL over 1 1/2 hours. A 10-drop set is used.

_____

3. You need to administer 350 mL of lactated ringers over 180 minutes using a 12-drop set.

_____

4. Figure how to administer 500 mL of normal saline over 2 hours using a 15-drop set.

_____

5. Using a 15-drop set, administer 100 mL of saline over 30 minutes.

_____

Objective

8.7 Determine the concentration of solutions.

A _solution_ is a liquid that has another substance, such as medication or minerals, dissolved in it. The substance that is dissolved in the liquid is called the _solute_. The liquid is called the _solvent_.

The **concentration of a solution** refers to the amount of the solute that has been dissolved in a specific amount of liquid. Concentrations are frequently noted by the use of percentages.

Example

If 2 parts of a mineral are placed in 100 parts of liquid, the concentration of the solution is 2:100. This could also be noted as 2/100, 0.02, or 2%.

SKILL SHARPENER

Indicate the ratio of solute to solvent in the following, first by using a ratio (x:100) and then by converting to a percentage (x%).

1. 4 parts of drug in 100 parts of liquid

_____ :100   _____ %

2. 12.5 parts of a mineral in 100 parts of liquid

_____ :100   _____ %

3. 50 parts of glucose in 100 parts water

_____ :100   _____ %

4. 10 parts of glucose in 100 parts water

_____ :100   _____ %

5. 9 parts of sodium chloride in 100 parts water

_____ :100   _____ %

PERCENT STRENGTH

Percent strength refers to the percentage of solvent in a given solute. For instance, if the medication order is for 10 mL of a 25% solution, first realize that the 25% refers to 25 parts of 100, noted as 25:100. Since you must give 10 mL of the solution, use proportions to figure how much of the drug or mineral would be mixed with the fluid to yield the desired solution.

The problem:

You are asked to administer 10 mL of a 25% solution.

Set up as:

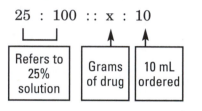

$$25 \ : \ 100 \ :: \ x \ : \ 10$$

| Refers to 25% solution | Grams of drug | 10 mL ordered |

Multiply the means. $25 : 100 :: x : 10$

$$100 \times x = 100x$$

Multiply the extremes. $25 : 100 :: x : 10$

$$25 \times 10 = 250$$

Set up as:

$$100x = 250$$

To solve for x, divide 100 into both sides.

$$100x \div 100 = 1x \text{ or } x$$

$$250 \div 100 = 2.5$$

Solution: x = 2.5

Therefore, mix 2.5 grams of drug in 10 mL to yield a 25% solution.

SKILL SHARPENER

How much of the solvent (drug or mineral) must be given to attain the following solutions? Figure using proportions and show your work.

1. 10 mL of a 6% solution _____

2. 75 mL of a 9% solution _____

3. 15 mL of a 35% solution _____

4. 150 mL of a 10% solution _____

5. 120 mL of a 0.9% solution. _____

Objective

8.8 Calculate medication dosages using proportions.

Every day, health care professionals calculate medication dosages in an effort to administer the correct amount of medication for the best therapeutic effect. Though there are a number of ways that medication doses are figured, proportions will be used here. By using critical thinking skills, proportions will help you to solve a vast number of problems.

The problem:

> You are asked to administer 40 mg of furosemide.
> It is packaged 10 mg/mL in an 8 mL ampule.

Set up as:

> 40 mg : x mL :: 10 mg : 1 mL

Multiply the means. 40 : x :: 10 : 1

> $x \times 10 = 10x$

Multiply the extremes. 40 : x :: 10 : 1

> $40 \times 1 = 40$

Set up as:

> $10x = 40$

To solve for x, divide both sides by 10.

> $10x \div 10 = 1x$ or x

> $40 \div 10 = 4$

Solution: x = 4 mL

Therefore, administer 4 mL to deliver 40 mg of furosemide.

SKILL SHARPENER

In each of the following problems, use proportions to determine the volume of medication to be given.

1. You are asked to administer 60 mg of furosemide. It is packaged 10 mg/mL in an 8 mL ampule. How many mL do you administer?

   _____

2. Administer 0.65 mg of dexamethasone elixir. It is packaged 0.5 mg/mL. How many mL do you administer?

   _____

3. Lidocaine is available in an ampule with 100 mg in 5 mL of solution. How many mL do you give to administer 65 mg?

   _____

4. Lorazepam is supplied 2 mg/mL in a 1 mL vial. You need to administer 3 mg slow IV. How many mL do you give?

   _____

5. Lovastatin is supplied in 20 mg tablets. You are asked to administer 60 mg. How many tablets do you give?

   _____

6. Lovenox is packaged 120 mg/0.8 mL. How many mL do you give to administer 40 mg?

_____

7. Compazine is supplied 10 mg in a 2 mL vial. How many mL do you give to administer 2.5 mg?

_____

8. Tenormin is supplied 5 mg in 10 mL ampules. How may mL do you give to administer 5 mg?

_____

9. You are called upon to administer 8 units Pitocin. It is supplied in a 1 mL ampule that contains 10 units. How many mL do you administer?

_____

10. You need to administer 1 mg of epinephrine. It is packaged 10 mg/10 mL. How many mL do you administer?

_____

Objective

8.9 Convert medication dosages for home use.

Patients sometimes have to take medications at home. Health care professionals may be called upon to instruct patients how to convert measurements from the metric or apothecary system to the household system. For instance, a patient may be asked to take 5 mL of a cough elixir. As a health care professional, you should be able to instruct him or her to take 1 teaspoon (tsp) as an approximate equivalent.

The ability to assist patients in this way depends on:

- knowing metric/apothecary/household equivalents.

- being able to use proportions to make conversions as necessary.

- knowing the necessary terminology and abbreviations.

A listing of common abbreviations is included in Appendix B and equivalencies are noted in Appendix C.

SKILL SHARPENER

Using the household system of measurement, clearly write how much and how often the patient should take the medicine. Use Appendix B and Appendix C if necessary.

1. The prescription calls for the patient to take 15 mL of a cough syrup PO b.i.d.

   _____

   _____

   _____

2. The order calls for 1 fldr of an elixir PO q.i.d.

_____

_____

_____

3. Instruct the patient to take 25 mg PO q 4 hours prn nausea. The medicine is supplied in 25 mg tablets.

_____

_____

_____

4. The patient should take 240 mg PO qd until gone. The prescription says to dispense #14, 120 mg capsules.

_____

_____

_____

5. Take 1/150 gr SL prn chest pain. This medication comes packaged in 0.4 mg tablets.

_____

_____

_____

6. The doctor wants the patient to take gr ss PO t.i.d. The tablets are 10 mg.

_____

_____

_____

7. The doctor orders 0.5 g to take PO b.i.d. The capsules come in 250 mg strength.

_____

_____

_____

8. The patient must drink a substance before a test the following day. The patient should take 240 mL PO HS, then should be NPO until after the test.

_____

_____

_____

9. The patient should take 1 oz of medication PO pc.

_____

_____

_____

10. Direct the patient to take 2 dr PO q.o.d.

_____

_____

_____

CONCLUSION

Medication administration is an important responsibility that should not be taken lightly. Health care professionals must assure that patients receive the intended dose of the correct medicine by carefully interpreting orders, accurately calculating dosages, and unfalteringly administering the intended medication.

Attention to detail is imperative. Erroneously moving the decimal one place in either direction could result in administering one tenth or ten times the desired dose of a drug. Though calculating medication dosages may be a routine part of a typical day, the health care professional must remain alert and diligent to ensure accuracy.

SELF-ASSESSMENT **POST-TEST**

Label the components of this medication label.

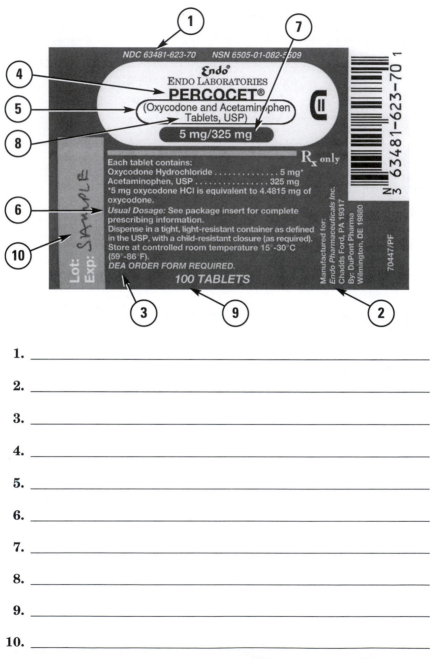

1. _____

2. _____

3. _____

4. _____

5. _____

6. _____

7. _____

8. _____

9. _____

10. _____

Label the components of this prescription.

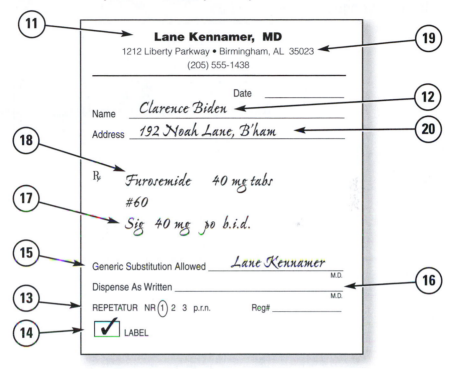

11. _____

12. _____

13. _____

14. _____

15. _____

16. _____

17. _____

18. _____

19. _____

20. _____

Determine the amount of solution remaining in each of the following syringes.

21. _____

22. _____

23. _____

24. _____

25. _____

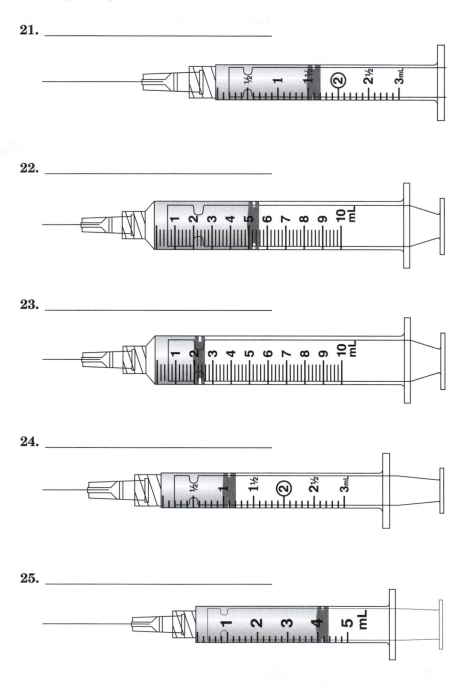

26. _____

27. _____

28. _____

29. _____

30. _____

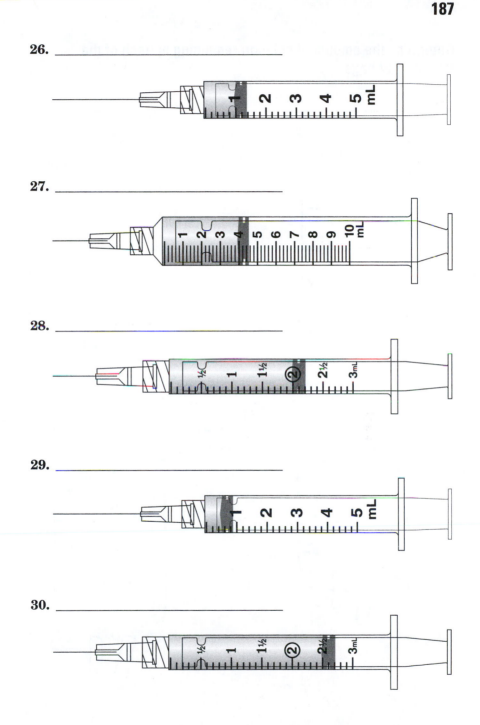

Determine the amount of solution remaining in each of the following IV bags.

31. _____

32. _____

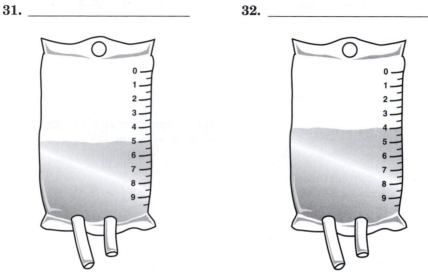

33. _____

34. _____

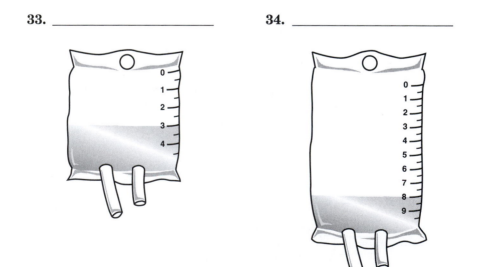

35. _____

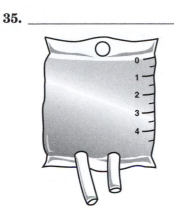

36. _____

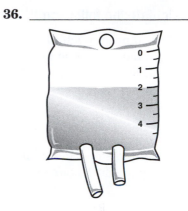

37. _____

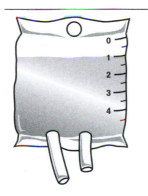

38. _____

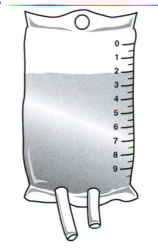

39. _____

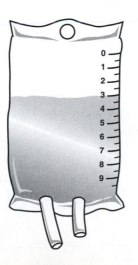

40. _____

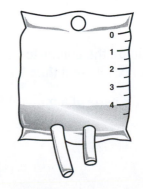

Calculate the following IV drip rates.

41. You need to administer 250 mL
of normal saline over a 3-hour
period using a 15-drop set.   _____

42. Administer 125 mL of lactated
ringers in 1 hour using a 12-drop set.   _____

43. Administer 750 mL of saline over
12 hours using a 10-drop set.   _____

44. You are asked to administer 300 mL
of fluid over 90 minutes using a
15-drop set.   _____

45. You need to administer 400 mL of
normal saline over a 2-hour period
using a 10-drop set.   _____

Indicate the solute-to-solvent ratio in the following, first by using a
ratio (x:100) and then by converting to a percentage (x%).

46. 8 parts of a mineral in 100 parts of liquid

_____ :100   _____ %

47. 12 parts of a drug in 100 parts of water

_____ :100   _____ %

48. 25 parts of glucose in 100 parts water

_____ :100   _____ %

49. 1.5 parts drug in 10 parts water

_____ :100   _____ %

50. 3 parts of a mineral in 100 parts water

_____ :100   _____ %

How much of the solvent (drug or mineral) must be given to attain the following solutions? Figure using proportions and show your work.

51. 12 mL of a 3% solution   _____

52. 200 mL of a 2% solution   _____

53. 30 mL of a 9% solution   _____

54. 5 mL of a 4% solution   _____

55. 10 mL of a 0.5% solution   _____

In each of the following, use proportions to determine the volume of medication to be given.

56. You must administer 75 mg of Lidocaine.
It is packaged in a prefilled syringe with
100 mg in 5 mL of solution.   _____

57. Epinephrine is packaged 1 mg/mL in a
10 mL vial. How many mL do you
administer if you wish to give 3 mg?   _____

58. A drug is packaged 0.5 mg per mL.
How many mL do you give if your
order is for 3.5 mg?   _____

59. You are asked to give 5 mg of Tenormin. It is supplied 1 mg/2 mL in a 10 mL ampule. _____

60. Oxytocin is packaged in a 1 mL ampule that contains 10 units. How many mL do you give when administering 6 units? _____

Using the household system of measurement, write in simple terms how much and how often the patient should take the prescribed medicine.

61. Take 1/200 gr SL prn chest pain. Tablets are supplied as 0.3 mg.

_____

_____

_____

62. The physician orders 0.75 g to take PO t.i.d. Capsules come in 250 mg strength.

_____

_____

_____

63. Direct the patient to take 240 mg PO b.i.d. until gone. The prescription says to dispense #42, 80 mg tablets.

_____

_____

_____

64. The physician orders 1 dr of solution b.i.d.

_____

_____

_____

65. Explain to the patient to take 2 dr of elixir PO q.i.d.

_____

_____

_____

Weights and Measures

LEARNING **OBJECTIVES**

After completing this chapter, the reader will be able to:

- **9.1** Read scales.
- **9.2** Convert between English and metric weight measurements.
- **9.3** Read an English (household) ruler.
- **9.4** Read a metric ruler.
- **9.5** Convert between English and metric length measurements.
- **9.6** Read a thermometer.
- **9.7** Convert between Fahrenheit and Celsius.
- **9.8** Determine body surface area.

KEY **TERMS**

- body surface area (BSA)
- Celsius
- Fahrenheit
- nomogram

INTRODUCTION

Health care professionals may need to convert English and metric measures. This includes converting from yards, feet, and inches to meters, centimeters, and millimeters and from Fahrenheit to Celsius and Celsius to Fahrenheit. This chapter will introduce the concepts necessary to perform these operations.

Objective

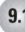 **9.1** Read scales.

Since some medication dosages are determined based on weight, it is important for health care professionals to accurately read scales and record weights. Read the scale as explained in Figure 9-1.

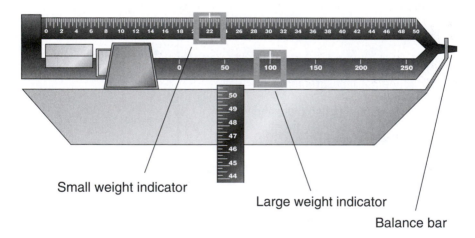

Small weight indicator

Large weight indicator

Balance bar

FIGURE 9-1 The weight shown on the upper and lower bars are added for the total weight.

Read the following scales.

1. _____

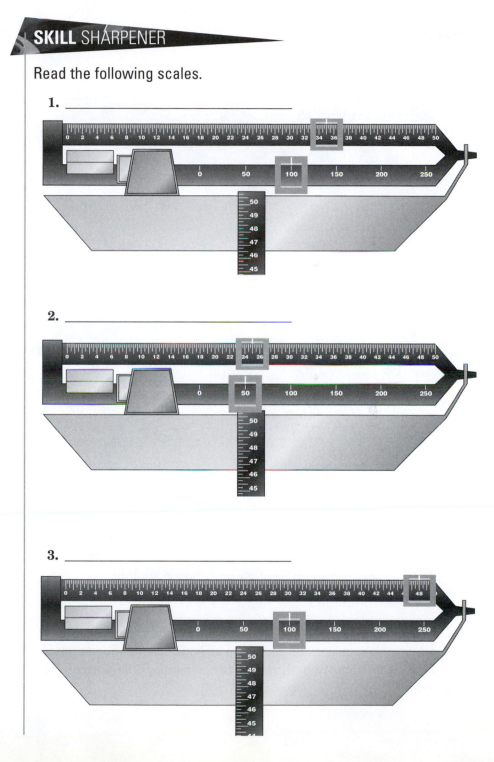

2. _____

3. _____

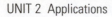

4. _____

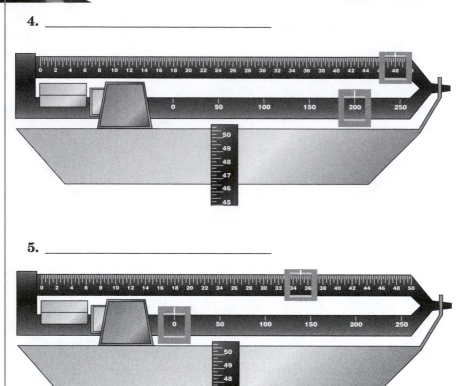

5. _____

Objective

 Convert between English and metric weight measurements.

To convert from English to metric weight measurements you must know the conversion formula, or equivalency. For example, 1 kilogram is roughly equivalent to 2.2 pounds. When converting from kilograms to pounds, multiply by 2.2.

Example: To convert 65 kilograms to pounds, multiply by 2.2.

Set up as:
$$65$$
$$\underline{\times\ 2.2}$$

Multiply.
$$65$$
$$\underline{\times\ 2.2}$$
$$130$$
$$\underline{130\ \ }$$
$$143.0$$

Solution: 65 kg = 143 lb

Conversely, to convert from pounds to kilograms, divide by 2.2.

Example: To convert 165 pounds to kilograms, divide by 2.2.

Set up as:

$$2.2\ \overline{)165}$$

Move decimals to right.

$$2.2\ \overline{)165.0}$$

Divide.
$$
\begin{array}{r}
75. \\
22\ \overline{)1650} \\
\underline{154} \\
110 \\
\underline{110} \\
0
\end{array}
$$

Solution: 165 lb = 75 kg

Convert the following from pounds to kilograms. Round to the nearest kilogram.

1. 220 lb _____

2. 175 lb _____

3. 40 lb _____

4. 12 lb _____

5. 195 lb _____

6. 155 lb _____

7. 90 lb _____

8. 120 lb   _____

9. 200 lb   _____

10. 6 lb   _____

Convert the following from kilograms to pounds. Round to the nearest pound.

11. 55 kg   _____

12. 100 kg   _____

13. 110 kg   _____

14. 22 kg   _____

15. 12 kg   _____

16. 90 kg   _____

17. 155 kg   _____

18. 80 kg   _____

19. 125 kg   _____

20. 130 kg   _____

Objective

9.3 Read an English (household) ruler.

Health care providers should be able to accurately read and record length measurements using both English and metric measurements. The English ruler uses inches and fractions of inches, which may be combined to form feet and/or yards. An example of an English ruler is illustrated in Figure 9-2.

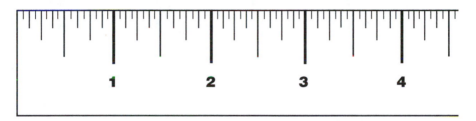

FIGURE 9-2 Household (English) ruler

To read the ruler, find the nearest inch mark to the left of the end of the item being measured. This is the number of inches. Then determine the fraction of an inch (if applicable) by determining where the end of the item being measured is. For example, this dropper measures 3 1/4 inches.

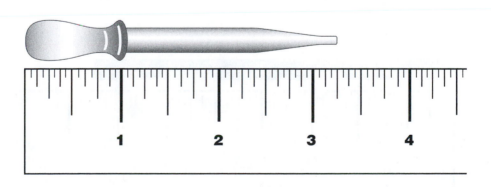

Record the length of the following bars.

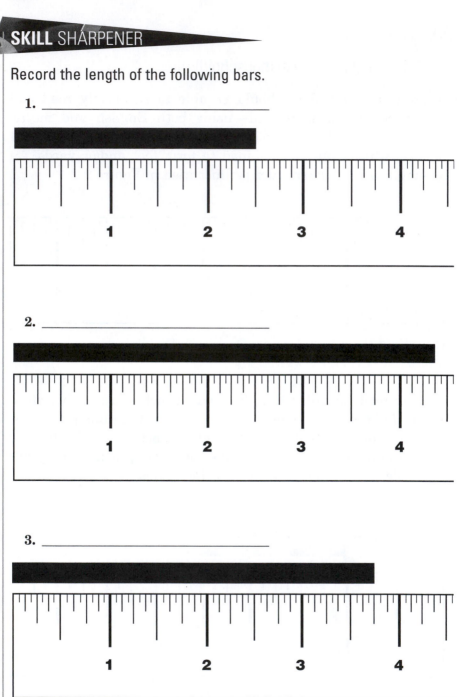

1. _____

2. _____

3. _____

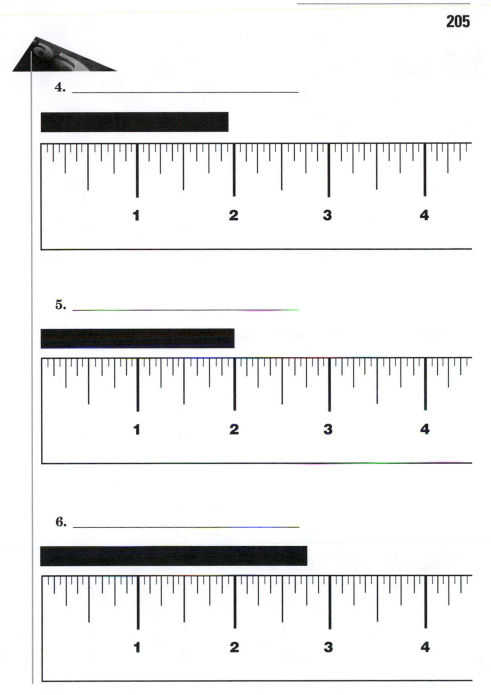

4. _____

5. _____

6. _____

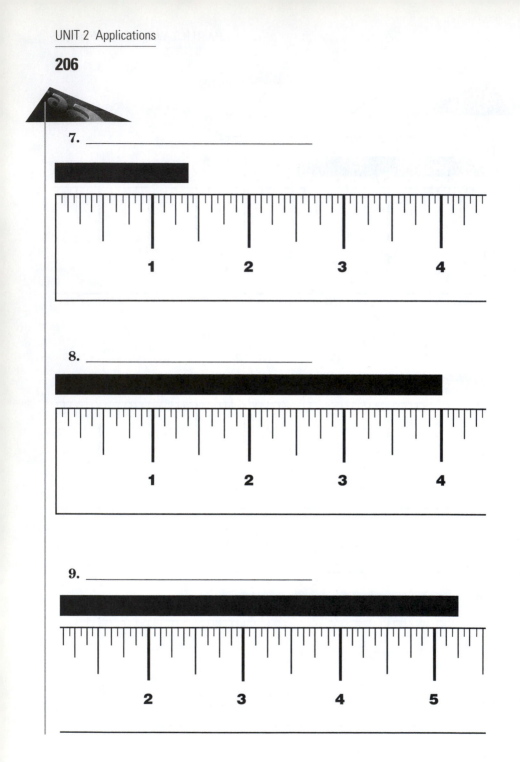

7. _____

8. _____

9. _____

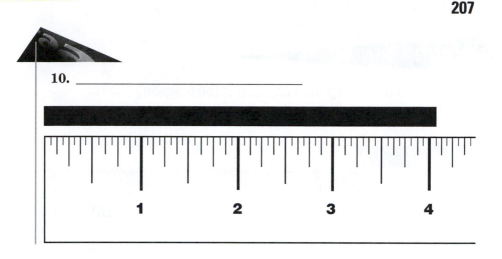

10. _____

Objective

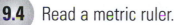

9.4 Read a metric ruler.

Because the metric system is based on tens, metric length measure is based on the meter. Lengths smaller than a meter are measured by tenths (decimeter), hundredths (centimeter), and thousandths (millimeter) of a meter, while lengths longer than a meter are measured by multiples of ten (dekameter), hundreds (hectometer), and thousands (kilometer).

The metric ruler is based on centimeters and millimeters. To read the metric ruler, find the mark closest to the item you are measuring. If it is a longer mark noted by a number, measure by centimeters. If it is a shorter mark, use millimeters. For example, the ruler shown in Figure 9-3 shows a reading of 2 centimeters, or 20 millimeters.

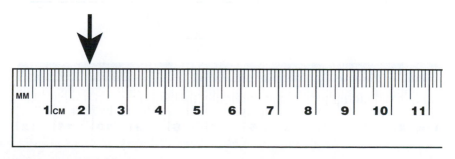

FIGURE 9-3 Metric ruler

SKILL SHARPENER

Note the lengths designated on each of the following rulers.

1. _____

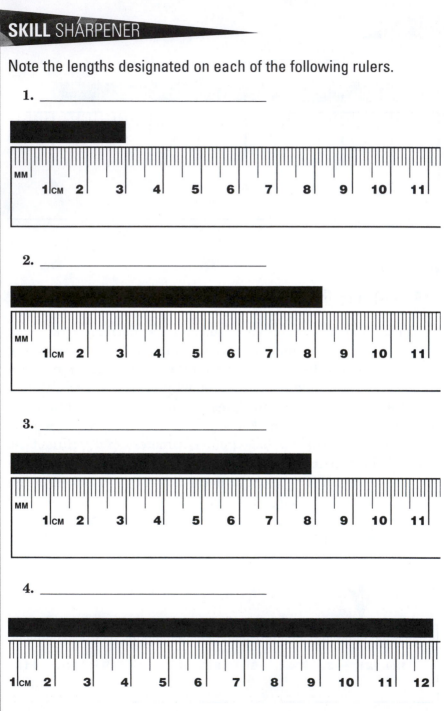

2. _____

3. _____

4. _____

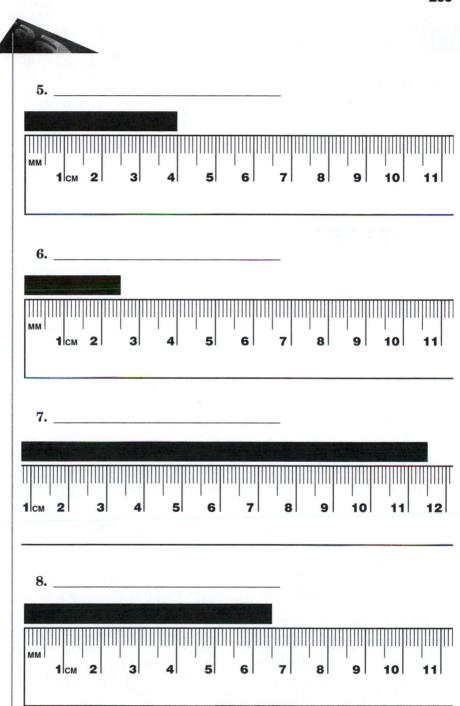

5. _____

6. _____

7. _____

8. _____

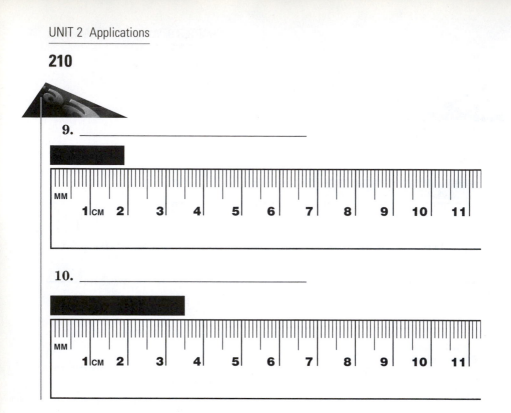

9. _____

10. _____

Objective

9.5 Convert between English and metric length measurements.

To convert between English and metric length measurements, you need to know the conversion factors or formulas. Key conversion formulas include the following.

1 inch	= 25.40 millimeters	= 2.54 centimeters
1 foot	= 12 inches	
1 yard	= 3 feet	
1 meter	= 39.37 inches	= 3.28 feet = 1.09 yards
1 dekameter	= 32.81 feet	
1 hectometer	= 328.08 feet	
1 kilometer	= 3280.08 feet	= 0.62 mile
1 millimeter	= 0.04 inch	
1 centimeter	= 0.39 inch	
1 decimeter	= 3.94 inches	

Example: Convert 3 meters to feet.

The problem:

3 meters = _____ feet

Set up as:

3 m : x ft :: 1 m : 3.28 ft

Multiply the means.   3 : x :: 1 : 3.28

x × 1 = 1x or x

Multiply the extremes.   3 : x :: 1 : 3.28

3 × 3.28 = 9.84

Solution: x = 9.84

Therefore, 3 meters = 9.84 feet.

SKILL SHARPENER

Convert the following feet to meters. Round to the nearest hundredth.

1. 10 feet   _____

2. 2 feet, 9 inches   _____

3. 9 feet, 3 inches   _____

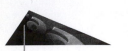

4. 4 1/2 feet

_____

5. 65 feet

_____

Convert the following meters to feet.

6. 19 meters

_____

7. 2.5 meters

_____

8. 13 meters

_____

9. 112 meters

_____

10. 84 meters

_____

Convert the following measurements to inches.

11. 3 feet _____

12. 2 feet _____

13. 2 1/2 feet _____

14. 5 feet, 3 inches _____

15. 1 1/2 meters _____

Objective

9.6 Read a thermometer.

Thermometers are instruments used to measure temperature. There are currently many types of thermometers available for use by health care professionals, including clinical glass thermometers, electronic thermometers, tympanic thermometers, and electronic thermometers. Figure 9-4 illustrates several types of thermometers.

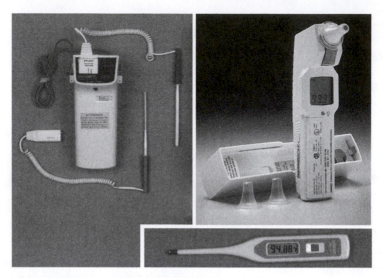

FIGURE 9-4 A variety of thermometers are available.

Most modern thermometers feature a digital readout, allowing the health care professional to simply read the temperature displayed in Hindu-Arabic numerals. Glass clinical thermometers, on the other hand, require some amount of skill and practice to secure an accurate reading. Figure 9-5 illustrates different types of glass clinical thermometers.

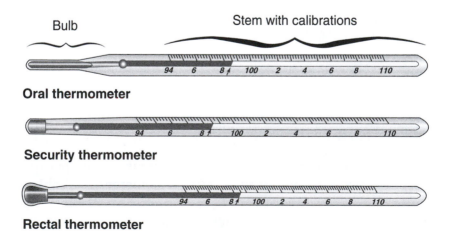

FIGURE 9-5 Types of clinical glass thermometers

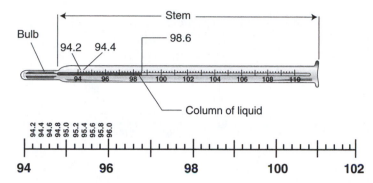

FIGURE 9-6 How to read a glass thermometer. This thermometer reads 98.6°F, the normal body core temperature.

Glass clinical thermometers are calibrated tubes that contain a column of colored liquid. Standard clinical thermometers start at 94°F with each long line indicating a one-degree elevation in temperature. Smaller lines indicate a 0.2°F variance in temperature. To read this type of thermometer, note the line at the end of the colored liquid and determine the number that the line represents. Figure 9-6 shows an example of how to read a clinical thermometer.

SKILL SHARPENER

Identify the temperatures illustrated on each of the following thermometers.

1. _____

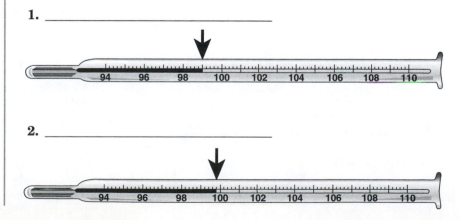

2. _____

3. _____

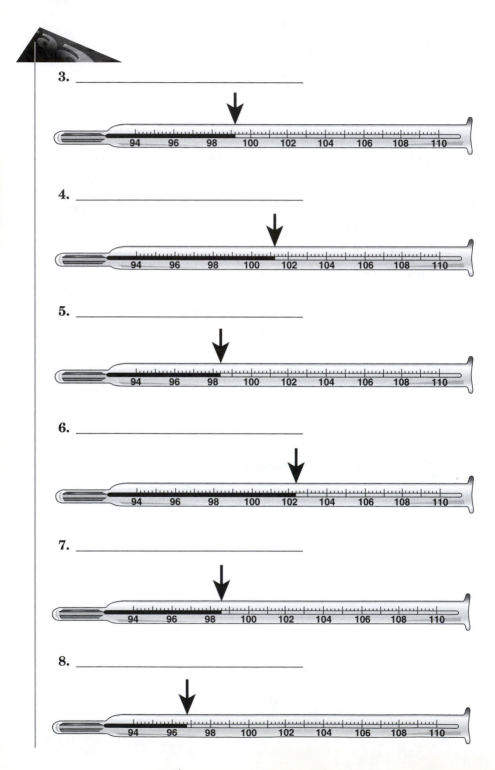

4. _____

5. _____

6. _____

7. _____

8. _____

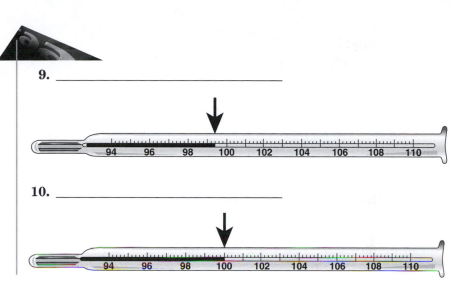

9. _____

10. _____

Objective

9.7 Convert between Fahrenheit and Celsius.

Fahrenheit is a thermometric scale in which water freezes at 32°F and boils at 212°F. **Celsius** is the international thermometric scale in which water freezes at 0°C and boils at 100°C. Sometimes it is necessary to convert between Fahrenheit (F) and Celsius (C) temperature measurements. To do this, use one of the following methods of conversion.

Fahrenheit to Celsius	Celsius to Fahrenheit
°F − 32 ÷ 1.8 = °C	°C × 1.8 + 32 = °F
or	or
°F − 32 × $\frac{5}{9}$ = °C	°C × $\frac{9}{5}$ + 32 = °F

Example: Convert 100°F to Celsius.

The problem:

$$100°F = \_\_\_\_\_ °C$$

Formula:

°F − 32 ÷ 1.8 = _____ °C

Set up as:

100°F − 32 ÷ 1.8 = _____ °C

Solve.

(100 − 32) ÷ 1.8 = _____ °C

68   ÷ 1.8 = 37.77°C

Solution: 100°F = 37.77°C

Example: Convert 100°C to Fahrenheit.

The problem:

100°C = _____ °F

Formula:

°C × 1.8 + 32 = _____ °F

Set up as:

100°C × 1.8 + 32 = _____ °F

Solve.

(100 × 1.8) + 32 = _____ °F

180   + 32 = 212°F

Solution: 100°C = 212°F

SKILL SHARPENER

Convert from Fahrenheit to Celsius.

1. 120°F   _____

2. 41°F   _____

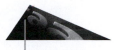

3. 99.6°F

_____

4. 101.3°F

_____

5. 102.9°F

_____

Convert from Celsius to Fahrenheit.

6. 32°C

_____

7. 87°C

_____

8. 12.9°C

_____

9. 43°C

_____

10. 55°C

_____

Objective

 9.8 Determine body surface area.

Body surface area (BSA) is used to determine drug dosages for infants and children, as well as a select group of adult patients. A mathematical estimate, expressed in square meters (m^2) of body surface area, is calculated based on the height and weight of the patient. Body surface area may be estimated through a mathematical calculation or by using a **nomogram**, a graphic image in which a straight line connects known values to find an unknown value. A nomogram for estimating body surface area is illustrated in Figure 9-7.

To use the nomogram, first determine the height and weight of the patient. Place a straight edge extending from the patient's weight in the right column to the patient's height in the left column. Now look at the place where the straight edge intersects the surface area (SA) column. This is the patient's estimated body surface area. If the patient is a child with normal height for his or her weight, the second column from the left (as illustrated in Figure 9-8) should be used.

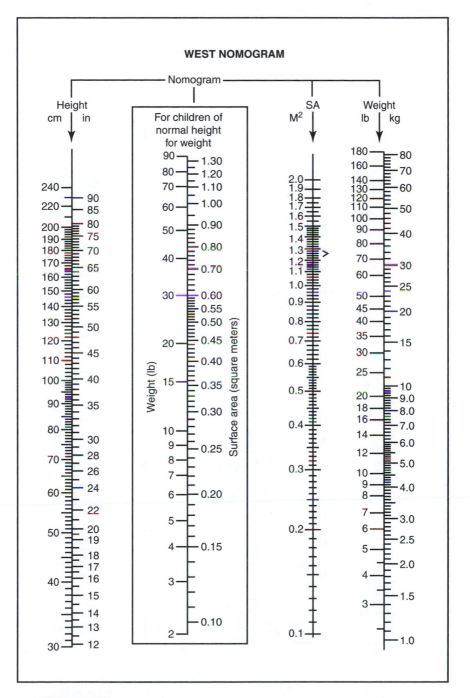

FIGURE 9-7 This nomogram may be used to estimate body surface area (BSA).

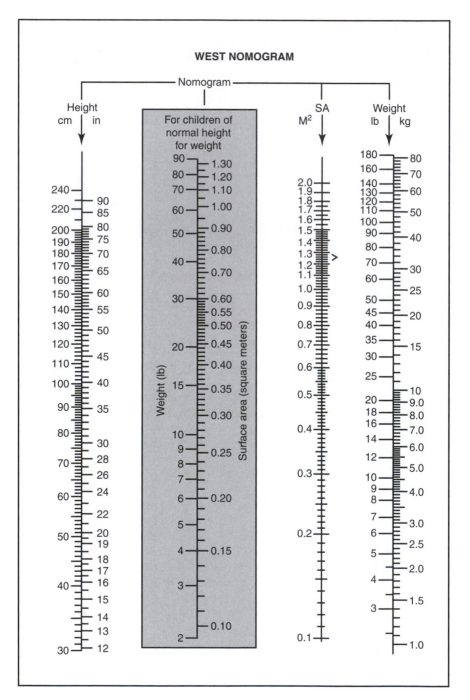

FIGURE 9-8 This nomogram may be used for children of normal height for their weight.

SKILL SHARPENER

Answer the following questions using the nomogram illustrated in Figure 9-7.

1. Your patient is a 7-year-old male who is 50 inches tall and weighs 50 pounds. What is his estimated BSA?

   _____

2. You need to find the BSA for a 10-year-old boy who is 55 inches tall and weighs 70 pounds. What is his estimated BSA?

   _____

3. Your patient weighs 40 kg and is 150 cm tall. What is the estimated BSA?

   _____

4. Your patient, who is of normal height for his weight, weighs 30 lb. What is his estimated BSA?

   _____

5. What is the estimated BSA for a female patient who weighs 65 pounds and is 60 inches tall?

   _____

6. What is the estimated BSA for a male patient who weighs 75 kg and is 70 inches tall?

   _____

7. What is the estimated BSA for a patient who is 190 cm and 60 kg?

_____

8. Determine the BSA for a patient who weighs 30 lb and is of normal height for her weight.

_____

9. What is the estimated BSA for a 10-lb infant?

_____

10. What is the estimated BSA for a patient of normal height for his weight of 25 lb?

_____

CONCLUSION

The ability of a health care provider to accurately read and document weights, lengths, and temperatures is vital to providing quality patient care. Accuracy is important, since weights and measurements affect medication dosages, and temperature is an important vital sign that may provide valuable insight into the patient's condition.

SELF-ASSESSMENT **POST-TEST**

Read the following scales.

1. _____

2. _____

3. _____

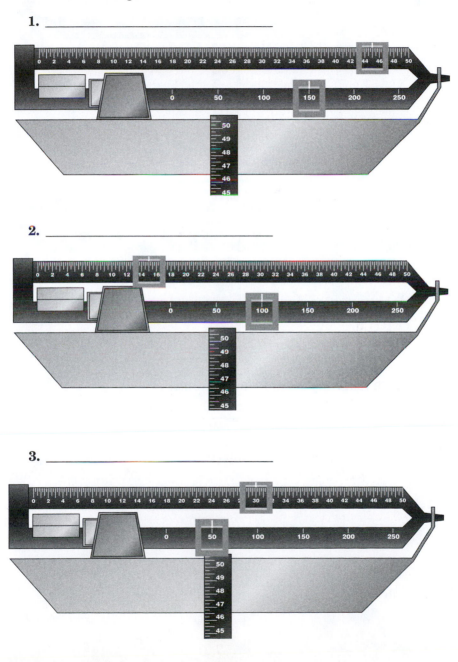

4. _____

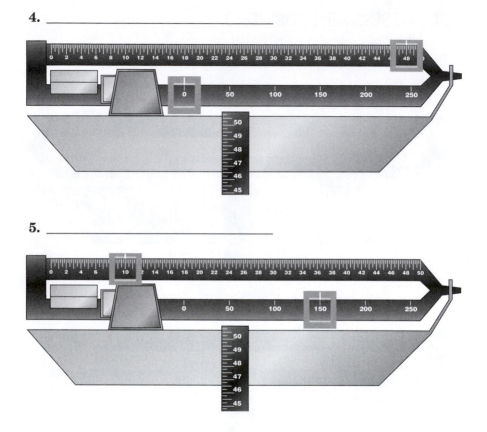

5. _____

Convert the following weights to kilograms.

6. 150 lb   _____

7. 222 lb   _____

8. 25 lb   _____

9. 39 lb   _____

10. 165 lb   _____

Convert kilograms to pounds.

11. 68 kg   _____

12. 9 kg   _____

13. 324 kg   _____

14. 75 kg   _____

15. 91 kg   _____

Record the lengths indicated on the following rulers.

16. _____

17. _____

18. _____

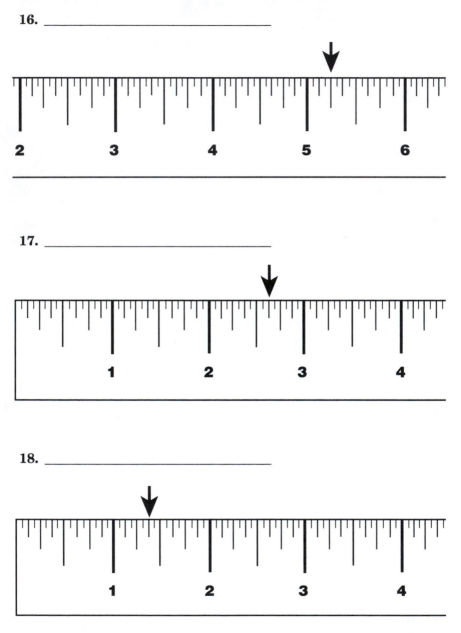

19. _____

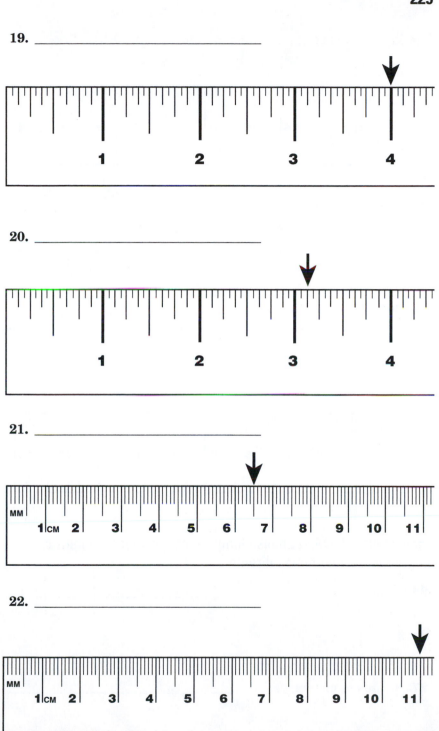

20. _____

21. _____

22. _____

23. _____

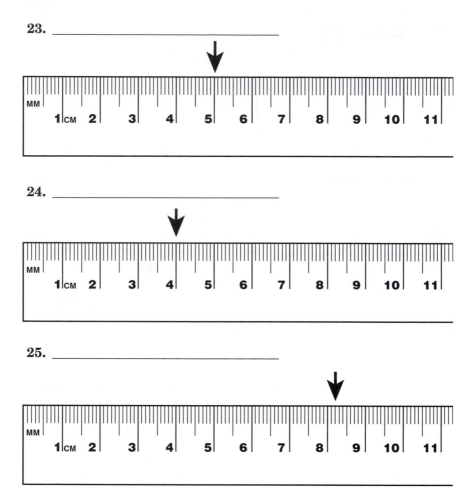

24. _____

25. _____

Convert the following English length measurements to metric length measurements as directed.

26. 17 feet to meters   _____

27. 9 yards to meters   _____

28. 6 feet to centimeters _____

29. 4 inches to centimeters _____

30. 2 1/2 inches to millimeters _____

Convert metric length measurements to English length measurements.

31. 3 meters to feet _____

32. 12 meters to feet _____

33. 33 meters to feet _____

34. 45 cm to inches _____

35. 575 mm to inches _____

Read the temperatures on the following thermometers.

36. _____

37. _____

38. _____

39. _____

40. _____

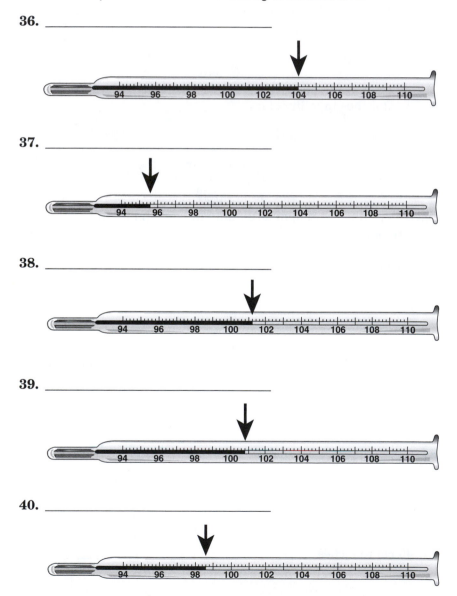

Convert the following temperatures from Fahrenheit to Celsius.

41. 98.6°F _____

42. 78°F _____

43. 102°F _____

44. 55°F _____

45. 1,250°F _____

Convert the following temperatures from Celsius to Fahrenheit.

46. 12°C _____

47. 34°C _____

48. 55°C   _____

49. 22°C   _____

50. 118°C   _____

Determine the estimated body surface area (BSA) for the following patients.

51. 35-lb child of normal height for her weight

_____

52. 7-lb infant of normal height for his weight

_____

53. 60-lb child of normal height for her weight

_____

54. 71-inch patient who weighs 80 kg

_____

55. 50-cm patient who weighs 5 kg

_____

Measuring Intake and Output

LEARNING **OBJECTIVES**

After completing this chapter, the reader will be able to:

10.1 Define intake and output.

10.2 Accurately measure urinary output.

10.3 Determine total daily output.

10.4 Determine intake by estimating.

10.5 Discover fluid imbalances by comparing intake and output.

KEY **TERMS**

- dehydration
- intake
- output
- overhydration

INTRODUCTION

Health care professionals monitor fluid intake and output in an effort to maintain fluid balance. It is important that intake and output be carefully measured and recorded so that imbalances are recognized and corrected early. Mathematical skills, including addition and estimating, are important in monitoring for fluid balance.

Objective

10.1 Define intake and output.

Intake refers to anything that goes into the body, either by mouth or intravenously. **Output** refers to liquid that is removed from the body. It is important that intake and output be balanced to prevent **dehydration**, or fluid deficit, and **overhydration**, or fluid excess.

Objective

10.2 Accurately measure urinary output.

Under several circumstances, urinary output should be measured to help determine the balance between intake and output. Often, health care professionals must measure urine in a graduated container or in a urinary catheter drainage bag. It is important that these measurements be taken and recorded accurately so that health care professionals recognize fluid imbalances and prescribe appropriate actions should imbalances occur.

To measure urinary output in a graduated container (Figure 10-1), place the container on a level surface and read the measurement at the nearest line.

To measure urinary output in a urinary bag (Figure 10-2), read the container at the nearest line.

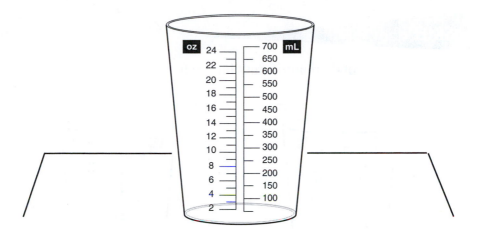

FIGURE 10-1 Place the graduated container on a flat surface for an accurate reading.

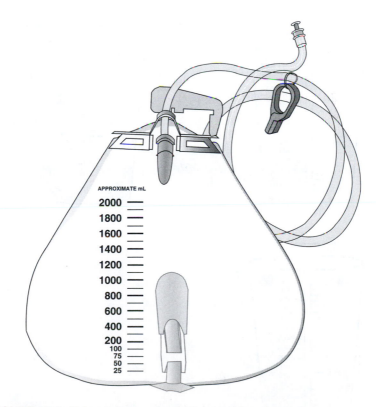

FIGURE 10-2 Urinary bags should be read level.

Determine the total urinary output for each container.

1. _____

2. _____

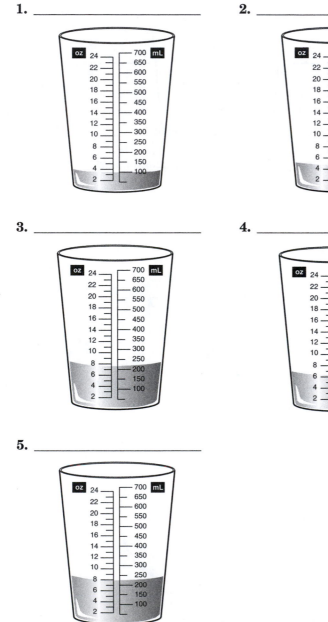
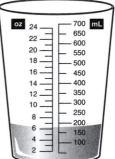

3. _____

4. _____

5. _____

6. _____

7. _____

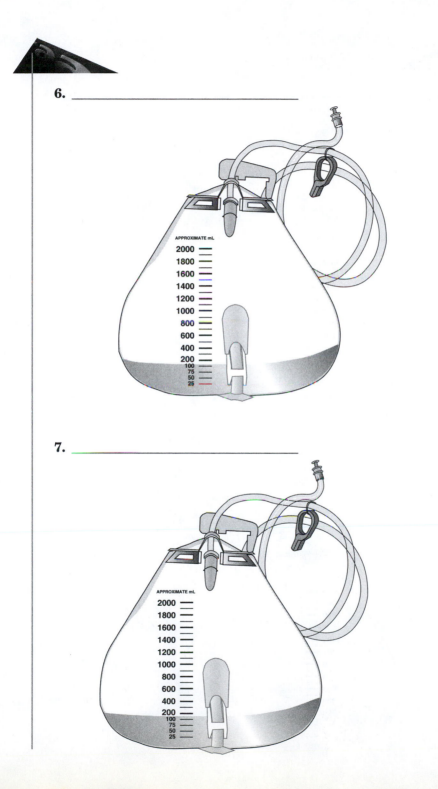

8. _____

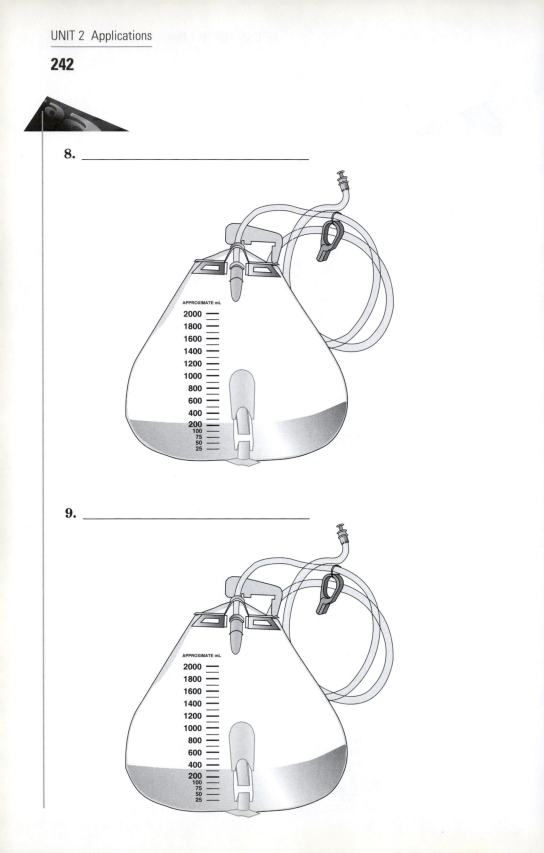

9. _____

10. _____

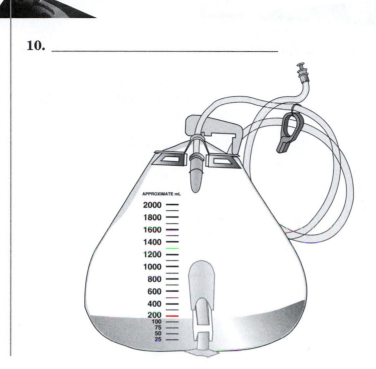

Objective

10.3 Determine total daily output.

The total daily output is the amount of fluid excreted from the body during a 24-hour period. Normally, this total daily output should be approximately the same as the total daily intake and should be in the range of approximately 1,500–2,000 mL.

Add the following recordings of output to determine the total daily output.

1. 1,000 mL of urine, 300 mL of vomitus, and 500 mL of drainage

_____

2. 1,500 mL of urine, 200 mL of drainage

_____

3. 2,000 mL of urine, 120 mL of vomitus

_____

4. 1,900 mL of urine, 200 mL of drainage, and 300 mL of vomitus

_____

5. Urine outputs of 350, 300, 250, 250, 350, and 250 mL

_____

6. Urine outputs of 400, 350, 400, 345, 255, and 400 mL and 300 mL of vomitus

   _____

7. Urine outputs of 300, 200, 225, 175, 300, 245, and 300 mL and 400 mL of drainage

   _____

8. Drainage of 200 mL and urinary output totaling 1,900 mL

   _____

9. Vomitus totaling 400 mL and urinary output totaling 1,300 mL

   _____

10. 2,000 mL of urine, 100 mL of drainage, and 200 mL of vomitus

   _____

Objective

10.4 Determine intake by estimating.

Since the health care professional may need an estimate of input to determine fluid balance, it is helpful to be able to estimate intake based on serving sizes and the amount the patient has eaten. To make this task easier, several estimation guides similar to the following exist.

Coffee/tea cup	8 oz = 240 mL
Glass	8 oz = 240 mL
Water carafe	16 oz = 480 mL
Foam cup	8 oz = 240 mL
Soup bowl	6 oz = 180 mL
Gelatin	1 serving = 130 mL
Ice chips	4 oz glass = 120 mL

SKILL SHARPENER

Estimate the amount of intake based on the following.

1. one glass of milk and 1/2 cup of coffee

_____

2. 1 cup of gelatin and 1/2 glass of orange juice

_____

3. 2 cups of gelatin, 2 cups of coffee, and 1/2 glass of tea

_____

4. 8 glasses of water, 3 glasses of milk, and 3 servings of gelatin

_____

5. 1/2 cup of coffee, 1/2 glass of juice, 4 glasses of tea, and 2 glasses
   of water

_____

Objective

10.5 Discover fluid imbalances by comparing intake
and output.

By comparing total daily intake and total daily output, the
health care provider determines if fluid imbalances exist. Early
recognition of imbalances helps to prevent dehydration or overhydration of the hospitalized or institutionalized patient.

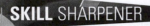

SKILL SHÁRPENER

Determine the fluid balance or imbalance of the following patients.

1. Mr. Genheim had a total fluid intake of 1,900 mL and a total fluid output of 1,850 mL.

_____

2. Mrs. Reed drank six glasses of water and ate four servings of gelatin. Her output includes urine output of 250 mL, 200 mL, 300 mL, 275 mL, 200 mL, and 295 mL.

_____

3. Mrs. Ahsirt had a total fluid intake of 2,000 mL and a total fluid output of 2,000 mL.

_____

4. Mr. Jones drank 6 glasses of water, 3 glasses of juice, 2 cups of coffee, 2 cups of soup, and 3 servings of gelatin. What should his output be to achieve fluid balance?

_____

5. Ms. Benjamin ate 3 cups of soup, 3 servings of gelatin, and drank 4 glasses of tea and 3 glasses of juice. To achieve fluid balance, what should Ms. Benjamin's output be?

_____

CONCLUSION

Mathematical skills are important in determining fluid intake, output, and balance. The skills of addition and comparison are vital in assuring that the health care professional is able to keep a close watch on fluid balance.

SELF-ASSESSMENT **POST-TEST**

Determine the amount of fluid in each of the following containers.

1. _____

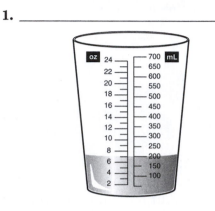

2. _____

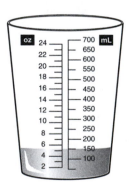

3. _____

4. _____

5. _____

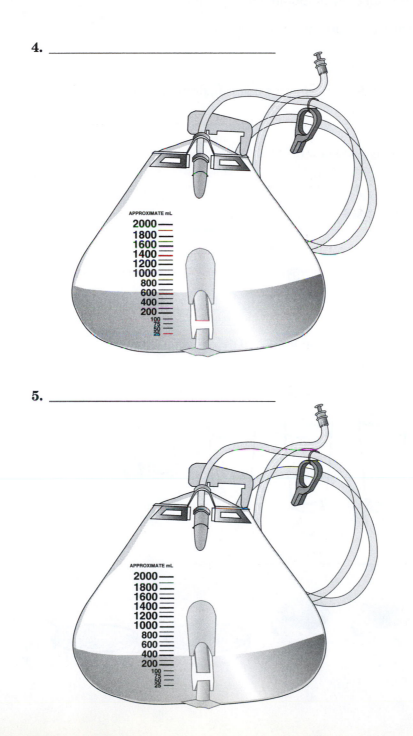

Find the total daily output in each of the following.

   6. urine 1,800 mL, drainage 300 mL

   _____

   7. urine 2,000 mL, vomitus 350 mL, drainage 200 mL

   _____

   8. drainage 600 mL, urine 1,200 mL

   _____

   9. vomitus 800 mL, urine 850 mL

   _____

  10. drainage 500 mL, urine 1,900 mL

   _____

Estimate the amount of intake, in mL, based on each of the following.

  11. _____

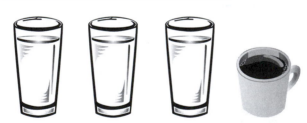

  12. _____

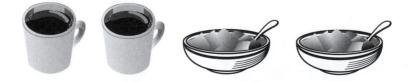

13. _____

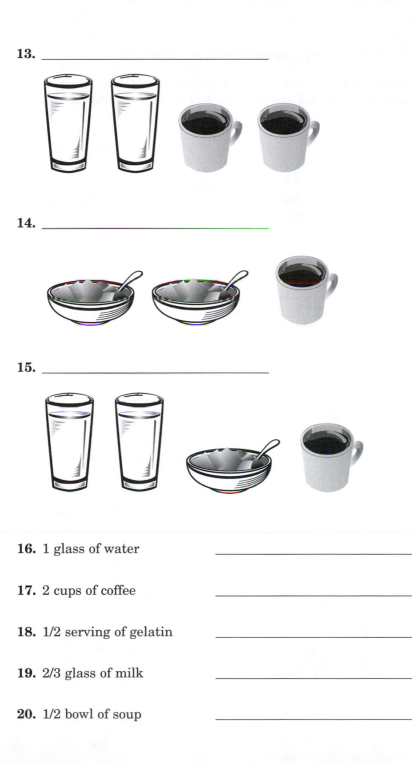

14. _____

15. _____

16. 1 glass of water   _____

17. 2 cups of coffee   _____

18. 1/2 serving of gelatin   _____

19. 2/3 glass of milk   _____

20. 1/2 bowl of soup   _____

Determine the balance between intake and output.

21. A patient had a total intake of 2,000 mL yesterday. Output included 1,500 mL of urine and 400 mL of fluid from drainage.

_____

22. Your patient had a total daily output of 1,800 mL. According to her intake chart, she drank 6 glasses of water, 1/2 cup of coffee, 2 glasses of tea, and 2 servings of gelatin.

_____

23. The resident in an extended care facility had a total intake of 2,200 mL and output of 2,000 mL urine and 250 mL vomitus.

_____

24. A patient had a daily output of 2,500 mL. According to records, he drank 2 glasses of water, 3 cups of coffee, 4 glasses of tea, and 1 1/2 servings of gelatin.

_____

25. The patient had a daily intake of 1,900 mL and an urinary output as follows: 150 mL, 250 mL, 200 mL, 200 mL, 350 mL, 150 mL, 350 mL, and 200 mL.

_____

This unit provides a set of resources that will be helpful not only for class, but also in real life. Knowledge of abbreviations will help save time and assure consistency with other health care professionals, while the equivalency and conversion charts will serve as helpful references both in school and in clinical practice.

The glossary includes all the key terms listed as bold in the text and will serve as a reference for many years. Helpful charts and tables are also provided as a handy reference.

UNIT

3

Additional Learning Resources

Resources

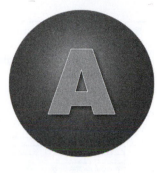

MULTIPLICATION TABLE

X	1	2	3	4	5	6	7	8	9	10	11	12
1	1	2	3	4	5	6	7	8	9	10	11	12
2	2	4	6	8	10	12	14	16	18	20	22	24
3	3	6	9	12	15	18	21	24	27	30	33	36
4	4	8	12	16	20	24	28	32	36	40	44	48
5	5	10	15	20	25	30	35	40	45	50	55	60
6	6	12	18	24	30	36	42	48	54	60	66	72
7	7	14	21	28	35	42	49	56	63	70	77	84
8	8	16	24	32	40	48	56	64	72	80	88	96
9	9	18	27	36	45	54	63	72	81	90	99	108
10	10	20	30	40	50	60	70	80	90	100	110	120
11	11	22	33	44	55	66	77	88	99	110	121	132
12	12	24	36	48	60	72	84	96	108	120	132	144

HEIGHT AND WEIGHT CHARTS

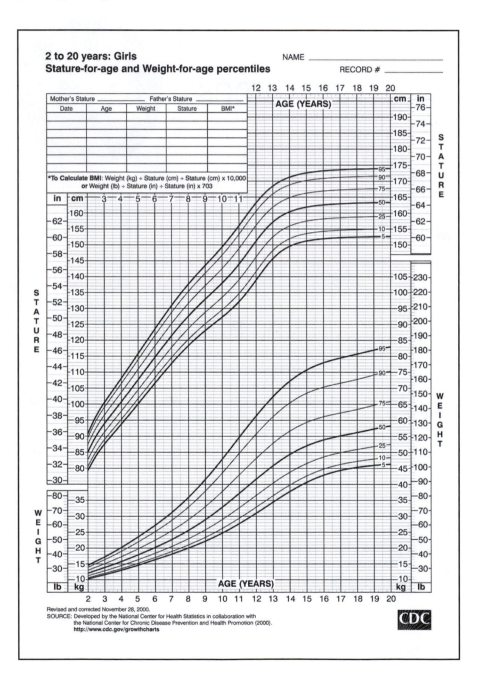

2 to 20 years: Girls
Stature-for-age and Weight-for-age percentiles

NAME _____

RECORD # _____

*To Calculate BMI: Weight (kg) ÷ Stature (cm) ÷ Stature (cm) x 10,000
or Weight (lb) ÷ Stature (in) ÷ Stature (in) x 703

Revised and corrected November 28, 2000.
SOURCE: Developed by the National Center for Health Statistics in collaboration with
the National Center for Chronic Disease Prevention and Health Promotion (2000).
http://www.cdc.gov/growthcharts

CDC

HEIGHT AND WEIGHT CHARTS *(continued)*

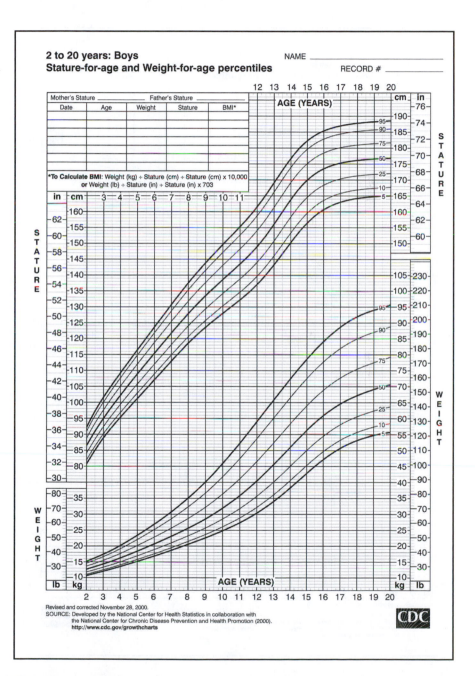

2 to 20 years: Boys
Stature-for-age and Weight-for-age percentiles

NAME _____

RECORD # _____

Mother's Stature _____ Father's Stature _____

Date	Age	Weight	Stature	BMI*

*To Calculate BMI: Weight (kg) ÷ Stature (cm) ÷ Stature (cm) x 10,000
or Weight (lb) ÷ Stature (in) ÷ Stature (in) x 703

Revised and corrected November 28, 2000.
SOURCE: Developed by the National Center for Health Statistics in collaboration with
the National Center for Chronic Disease Prevention and Health Promotion (2000).
http://www.cdc.gov/growthcharts

CDC

PEDIATRIC GROWTH CHARTS

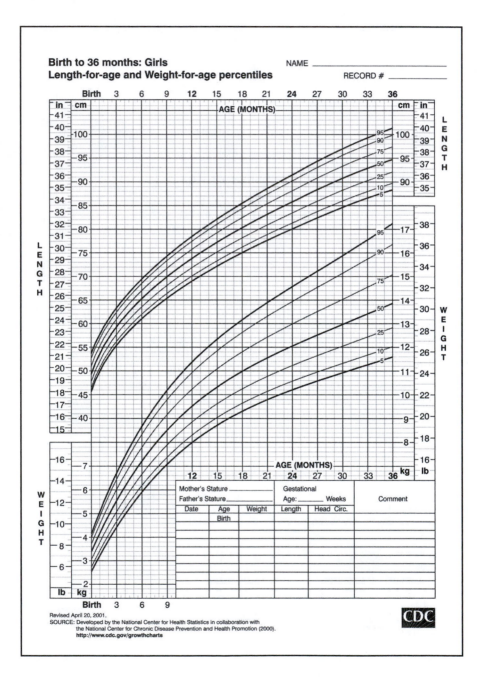

Birth to 36 months: Girls
Length-for-age and Weight-for-age percentiles

NAME _____

RECORD # _____

Revised April 20, 2001.
SOURCE: Developed by the National Center for Health Statistics in collaboration with
the National Center for Chronic Disease Prevention and Health Promotion (2000).
http://www.cdc.gov/growthcharts

PEDIATRIC GROWTH CHARTS *(continued)*

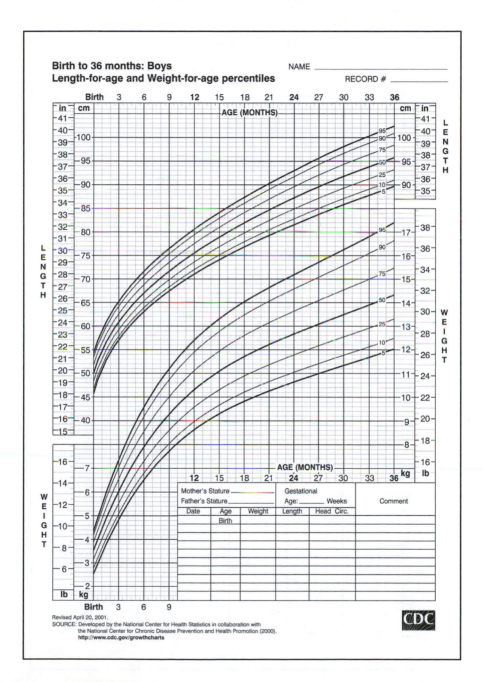

Birth to 36 months: Boys
Length-for-age and Weight-for-age percentiles

NAME _____

RECORD # _____

Revised April 20, 2001.
SOURCE: Developed by the National Center for Health Statistics in collaboration with
the National Center for Chronic Disease Prevention and Health Promotion (2000).
http://www.cdc.gov/growthcharts

BODY SURFACE AREA NOMOGRAM

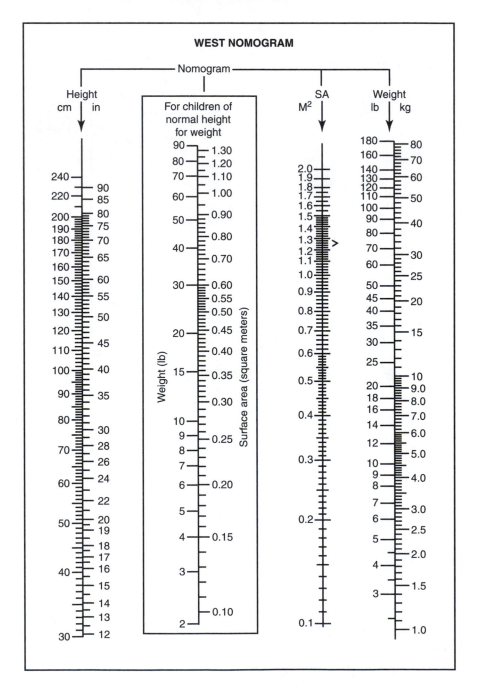

WEST NOMOGRAM

APPENDIX

Abbreviations

ā	of each		**elix.**	elixir
āā	of each		**F**	Fahrenheit
a.c.	before a meal		**fldr**	fluidram
alt. dieb.	every other day		**floz**	fluidounce
alt. hor.	every other hour		**g**	gram
alt. noc.	every other night		**gm**	gram
AM	morning		**gr**	grain
ap	before dinner		**gt**	drop
bib.	drink		**gtt**	drop
b.i.d.	twice a day		**h**	hour
b.i.n.	twice a night		**h.d.**	at bedtime
C	Celsius		**hr**	hour
c̄	with		**h.s.**	hour of sleep (bedtime)
cap.	capsule			
cc	cubic centimeter		**IM**	intramuscular
cm	centimeter		**inj**	injection
/d	per day		**I.U.**	international unit
dr	dram		**kg**	kilogram

L	liter		**q.2h**	every 2 hours
lb	pound		**q.3h**	every 3 hours
mcg	microgram (μ)		**q.4h**	every 4 hours
m	meter		**q.i.d.**	four times a day
m.	minim (℔)		**q.l.**	as much as desired
mEq	milliequivalent		**q.n.**	every night
mg	milligram		**q.o.d.**	every other day
mL	milliliter		**q.o.h.**	every other hour
mm	millimeter		**q.s.**	as much as is required
n.p.o.	nothing by mouth		**qt**	quart
non. rep.	not to be repeated		**rep.**	let it be repeated
o.d.	every day		**Rx**	take thou
o.h.	every hour		**s̄**	without
o.m.	every morning		**SC**	subcutaneously
o.n.	every night		**Sig.**	write on label
os	mouth		**SL**	sublingual
oz	ounce		**ss**	one half
p̄	after		**stat.**	immediately
p.c.	after meals		**T**	temperature
po	by mouth		**t.i.d.**	three times a day
PM	afternoon or evening		**t.i.n.**	three times a night
p.r.n.	as needed		**top.**	topically
pt	pint		**USP**	United States Pharmacopeia
q	every		**ut.dict.**	as directed
q.d.	every day			
q.h.	every hour			

APPENDIX

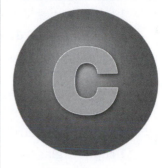

Equivalents

These equivalents are for your reference and provide an approximate, though generally accepted, measure. Frequently-used equivalents should be committed to memory.

LINEAR MEASURE

1 inch = 25.40 millimeters = 2.54 centimeters

1 foot = 12 inches

1 yard = 3 feet

1 meter = 39.37 inches = 3.28 feet = 1.09 yards

1 decameter = 32.81 feet

1 hectometer = 328.08 feet

1 kilometer = 3,280.08 feet = 0.62 mile

1 millimeter = 0.04 inch

1 centimeter = 0.39 inch

1 decimeter = 3.94 inches

WEIGHT

1 pound = 16 ounces	1 decigram = 1.54 grains
1 kilogram = 2.2 pounds	1 gram = 0.04 ounce
1 milligram = 0.02 grain	1 decagram = 0.35 ounce
1 centigram = 0.15 grain	1 hectogram = 3.53 ounces

LIQUID MEASURE

1 tablespoon = 3 teaspoons = 180 drops = 1/2 ounce

1 teaspoon = 60 drops = 1 fluidram

1 fluidounce = 6 teaspoons = 2 tablespoons = 8 fluidrams = 30 milliliters

1 quart = 2 pints = 32 ounces = 1000 milliliters = 4 glasses or cups

1 gallon = 4 quarts = 16 glasses or cups

1 cup = 1 glass = 8 ounces

1 pint = 500 milliliters = 2 glasses or cups = 16 fluidounces

1 medicine cup = 30 milliliters

1 grain = 60 milligrams

1 fluidram = 60 minims = 4 milliliters

1 minim = 1 drop

1 teacup = 6 ounces

1 milliliter = 15 minims

TIME

1 minute = 60 seconds

1 day = 24 hours

1 week = 7 days

1 year = 12 months

DRY MEASURE

1 grain = 60 milligrams

1 gram = 15 grains

1 tablespoon = 15 grams = 4 drams = 3 teaspoons

1 ounce = 30 grams

Glossary

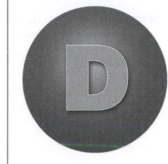

apothecary system—(Chapter 2) Measurement system that is used on a limited basis.

body surface area (BSA)—(Chapter 9) A mathematical estimate, expressed in square meters (m^2), used to calculate medication dosages, usually in children.

borrow—(Chapter 4) When subtracting, what you do when the digit you are subtracting is greater than the digit you are subtracting from. You must move, or borrow, a digit from the place to the immediate left, allowing you to subtract.

canceling—(Chapter 4) Finding the product of two fractions by reducing fractions.

Celsius—(Chapter 9) The international thermometric scale in which 0° is freezing and 100° is boiling.

common denominator—(Chapter 4) Denominators that are the same number.

common factor—(Chapter 4) A factor that belongs to two or more numbers.

concentration of a solution—(Chapter 8) The amount of solute that has been dissolved in a specific amount of fluid.

conversion—(Chapter 7) The act of changing from one system or measurement to another.

decimal—(Chapter 3) A fraction of a whole number whose denominators are multiples of 10.

dehydration—(Chapter 10) A fluid imbalance in which fluid is deficient.

denominator—(Chapter 4) The number of parts by which an item is divided. It is shown as the bottom number in a fraction.

drip rate—(Chapter 8) The rate in which the fluid drips from the intravenous bag into the intravenous line.

English system—(Chapter 2) Synonym for household system of measurement.

expiration date—(Chapter 8) The last date in which a medication should be used.

extremes—(Chapter 5) The end, or outside components, of a proportion.

factor—(Chapter 4) In multiplication, the numbers being multiplied.

Fahrenheit—(Chapter 9) The thermometric scale in which 32° is freezing and 212° is boiling.

fraction—(Chapter 4) A part of a whole.

generic name—(Chapter 8) Nonproprietary name of a medication.

greatest common factor (GCF)—(Chapter 4) The largest factor that two or more numbers have in common.

Hindu-Arabic system—(Chapter 1) A numerical system developed approximately 600 A.D. in India by the Hindus and brought to the Western world by the Arabs. It is sometimes referred to as the Arabic system.

household system—(Chapter 2) System of measurement that utilizes measuring devices that are readily available in most homes. Prescribed medications are frequently converted to household measures.

improper fraction—(Chapter 4) A fraction in which the numerator is greater than the denominator.

intake—(Chapter 10) That which is taken into the body.

KVO line—(Chapter 8) Keep vein open. Designation for intravenous drip rate that runs as a rate sufficient to keep a line open for medication administration.

least common denominator (LCD)—(Chapter 4) The lowest number into which all the denominators in a set can be divided.

least common multiple (LCM)—(Chapter 4) The smallest multiple that is shared by two or more numbers.

lot number—(Chapter 8) Internal reference number used by a manufacturer so that medications may be traced to the day and the batch in which they were manufactured.

macrodrip—(Chapter 8) Drip set commonly used for fluid replacement and/or to keep a route available for intra-venous medications; commonly available in 10, 12, or 15 drops per mL. Also referred to as a standard drip set.

means—(Chapter 5) The middle components of a proportion.

medication label—(Chapter 8) A label that contains important information to help the health care professional deliver the right medication to the patient. Components of the medication label include trade name, generic name, manufacturer, NDC number, dosage strength, drug form, usual adult dose, total amount enclosed, prescription warning, expiration date, and lot number.

metric system—(Chapter 2) A decimal system of weights and measures based on the meter, liter, and gram.

microdrip—(Chapter 8) Intravenous drip set used when volume must be limited. A microdrip set delivers one mL for every 60 drops of fluid that drips through the set.

mixed number—(Chapter 4) A combination consisting of a whole number and a fraction.

multiple—(Chapter 4) The product of a whole number multiplied by a whole number.

nomogram—(Chapter 9) A graphic image in which a straight line connects known values to find an unknown value; sometimes used to measure body surface area and children's height and weight.

numerator—(Chapter 4) The number of parts represented in the fraction. It is shown as the top number in the fraction.

numerical system—(Chapter 1) An organized system for counting.

output—(Chapter 10) Liquid that is excreted from the body.

overhydration—(Chapter 10) A fluid imbalance in which there is an excess of fluids.

percent (%)—(Chapter 6) A part of one hundred.

percent strength—(Chapter 8) Refers to the percentage of a solvent in a given solute.

piggyback—(Chapter 8) A medication infusion that is attached to an already existing (primary) IV line.

place value—(Chapter 3) The value of a digit specified by its location in relation to the decimal.

prescription—(Chapter 8) A medication order that a physician writes or telephones to a pharmacy.

proper fraction—(Chapter 4) A fraction in which the denominator is greater than the numerator.

proportion—(Chapter 5) An equation that states that two ratios are equal.

ratio—(Chapter 5) A comparison of numbers by division.

Roman numerals—(Chapter 1) An additive system created by ancient Romans. This system is thought to have evolved from tick marks on the ground and is still used on a limited basis today. Numbers are read by adding and/or subtracting a series of symbols.

syringe—(Chapter 8) Graduated cylindrical container that is used to administer precise amounts of medication.

terms—(Chapter 5) The numbers that are compared in a ratio.

TKO line—(Chapter 8) To keep open. Designation for intravenous drip rate that runs as a rate sufficient to keep a line open for medication administration.

trade name—(Chapter 8) The proprietary name of a medication, usually protected by a trademark.

uncommon denominator—(Chapter 4) Denominators that are not the same.

uncommon factor—(Chapter 4) Factors that are not common to two or more numbers.

whole number—(Chapter 4) Any of the set of nonnegative integers.

Final Summative Evaluation

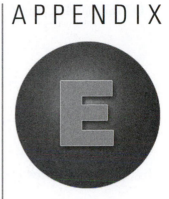

Answer each of the following problems.

You are asked to weigh and measure a new patient in your unit. When you weight Mrs. Ahsirt, you note the following reading.

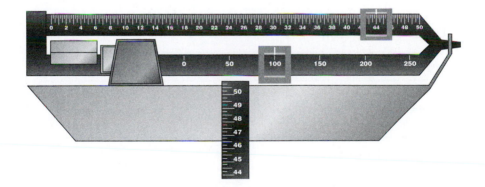

You note Mrs. Ahsirt's height on the rule below.

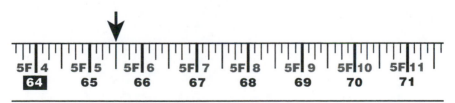

1. What is Mrs. Ahsirt's weight in pounds?

   _____

2. What is Mrs. Ahsirt's height in English measurement?

   _____

Mrs. Ahsirt's orders include the following:

MEDICATION	DOSAGE	ROUTE	FREQ
Cephalexin cap.	500 mg	PO	q6h

3. Check the box of the correct medications.

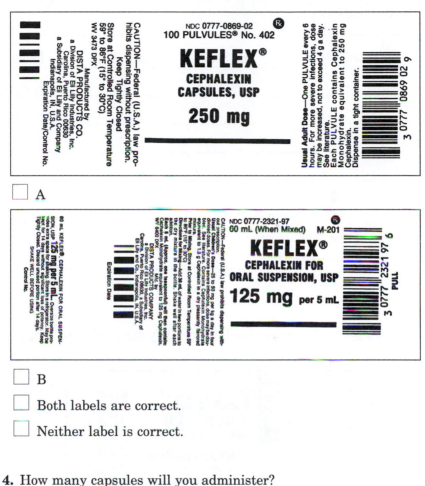

□ A

□ B

□ Both labels are correct.

□ Neither label is correct.

4. How many capsules will you administer?

_____

5. How frequently will this medicine be administered?

_____

6. What is the trade name of this medication?

_____

7. Who is the manufacturer of this medication?

_____

Another patient, Mr. Genheim, has the following order written on his chart.

MEDICATION	DOSAGE	ROUTE	FREQ
Furosemide	*80 mg*	*iv*	*non. rep.*

You locate the following medication in your medicine room.

Caution: Federal law prohibits dispensing without prescription.
Manufactured for:
HOECHST-ROUSSEL
Pharmaceuticals Inc.
Somerville, N.J. 08876
REG TM HOECHST AG
65604285

Lasix®
(furosemide)
Injection IM/IV
For Single Use Only
4 mL Vial
4 mL – 40 mg(10 mg/mL)

Store at controlled room temperature (59°–86°F).
Do not use if solution is discolored.

8. What is the trade name for this medicine?

_____

9. How many mL do you administer?

_____

10. How often will this dose be administered?

_____

A pharmacist receives the following prescription for Mrs. Brown.

Lane Kennamer, MD
1212 Liberty Parkway • Birmingham, AL 35023
(205) 555-1438

_____

Date *March 7, 2004*

Name *Jane Brown*

Address *401 5th St., Birmingham, AL*

℞ *Fexofenadine Hcl*
60 mg tabs
#60
Sig 60 mg po b.i.d.

Generic Substitution Allowed _____
                                                        M.D.
Dispense As Written ___*Lane Kennamer*_____
                                                        M.D.
REPETATUR NR 1 2 3 p.r.n.   Reg# *3462*_____

[✓] LABEL

11. How many tablets are prescribed?

_____

12. If the patient takes this medicine as directed, how many days will this prescription last?

_____

13. This medicine should be stored at a temperature of between 20°C to 25°C. In Fahrenheit, what temperature range should this medicine be kept?

_____

Your patient has consumed the following:

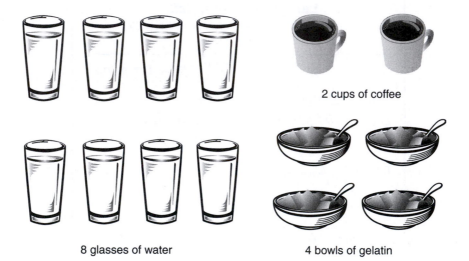

2 cups of coffee

8 glasses of water   4 bowls of gelatin

14. Estimate this patient's intake.

_____

15. What would you expect this patient's output to be?

_____

You are asked to start an intravenous line on Mr. Linden. The physician asks you to administer 600 mL of lactated ringers over 4 hours.

16. Circle the most appropriate drip set.

   a. Microdrip (60 drop set)

   b. Macrodrip (10 drop set)

17. Based on the drip set that you chose in question 17, at what rate would you run the IV?

_____

18. Your unit stocks 500 mL bags of lactated ringers. At the ordered rate, how quickly will the 500 mL bag empty?

_____

19. What percentage of the second 500 mL bag will be administered to the patient to comply with the physician's orders?

_____

20. You are asked to administer Lorazepam, 3mg to your patient. Lorazepam is supplied in 0.5 mg, 1 mg, and 2 mg tablets. What combination of these tablets would you administer to attain the ordered dose?

_____

Your patient's prescription calls for Amoxapine 100 mg t.i.d. Amoxapine is supplied in 50 mg tablets.

21. How often do you direct the patient to take his medicine?

_____

22. How many tablets will the patient take to meet his 100 mg dose?

_____

23. After three days, the patient calls you to inform you that he believes he has missed one or more doses of his medicine. Assuming that he has taken the appropriate number of doses each of the three days since his prescription was filled, how many tablets should the patient have taken so far?

_____

24. You are asked to administer 4,000 units of Botulinum Toxin, Type B to your patient. This medication is supplied 5,000 units/mL. How many mL will you administer?

_____

25. You need to administer 5 mg/kg of Bretylium tosylate to your patient, who weighs 195 lbs. Bretylium is supplied 50 mg/mL. How many mL will you administer?

_____

ANSWERS TO QUESTIONS

CHAPTER 1 NUMERICAL SYSTEMS

Objective 1.2 Skill Sharpener

1. 26
2. 651
3. 601
4. 1,150
5. 138
6. 1,965
7. 2,000
8. 3,540
9. 24
10. 660

Objective 1.3 Skill Sharpener

1. CVL
2. MMMCDXX
3. CCCXII
4. CDLIII
5. MCCCXCIV
6. MCCL
7. XXXVIII
8. CCCLXV
9. MMMCCXVII
10. CCCXXXIII

Post-Test

1. 4
2. 12
3. 1,154
4. 5
5. 8
6. 36
7. 19
8. 190
9. 1,983
10. 1,965
11. MMIII
12. XIV
13. XCVIII
14. MMMCDLVI
15. CCXXXI
16. DCCXCVIII
17. CDLXV
18. II
19. LXXII
20. CXII

CHAPTER 2   MEASUREMENT SYSTEMS

Objective 2.2 Skill Sharpener

Apothecary System of Weight

1. 3 gr
2. $\frac{2}{3}$ ʒ
3. 8 oz or 8 ʒ
4. 4 lb
5. $\frac{1}{200}$ gr
6. $\frac{1}{2}$ ʒ or ʒ ss

7. 3 oz or 3 ℥
8. 2 lb
9. 2 lb 11 oz or 2 lb 11 ℥
10. ½ gr or gr Ss

Apothecary System of Volume

1. 4 ℳ or 4 m
2. 1 fldr or 1 f℥
3. 3 floz
4. ½ pt
5. 2 qt
6. 3 gal.
7. 2 m or 2 ℳ
8. 8 floz
9. 5 fldr or 5 f℥
10. 2½ gal

Objective 2.4 Skill Sharpener

Prefixes

1. $\frac{1}{10}$ or 0.1
2. 10
3. 1,000
4. $\frac{1}{1000000}$ or 0.000001
5. $\frac{1}{1000}$ or 0.001
6. 100
7. $\frac{1}{100}$ or 0.01

Metric Units of Measure

	Measure of	Multiple or fraction
1.	length	fraction
2.	volume	fraction
3.	length	multiple
4.	volume	fraction
5.	weight	fraction
6.	volume	multiple
7.	volume	fraction
8.	weight	multiple
9.	weight	multiple
10.	length	fraction

Post-Test

1. A
2. C
3. B

4. C
5. A
6. B
7. A
8. B
9. A
10. B

CHAPTER 3 DECIMALS

Objective 3.2 Skill Sharpener

1. 12③.00
2. 9⑧.37
3. 2①.938
4. 3⑨.09
5. 2,22②.222
6. 56⑨987
7. 884⓪9
8. 9,292⑦7382
9. 478,333⑨29
10. 993⑨09
11. 8,437.0③03
12. 12,267.0⓪9772
13. 487.0⑨32
14. 9.3④1876
15. 4,576.8⑧8
16. 637,367.89⑥9
17. 988,989.43④233
18. 895.20⑨0
19. 57,847.05④9
20. 0009.00⓪09

Objective 3.3 Skill Sharpener

1. 175.98
2. 7,043.742
3. 99,349.67
4. 33.90
5. 17.7631

Objective 3.4 Skill Sharpener

1. >
2. <
3. >

4. >
5. <
6. <
7. =
8. <
9. =
10. =

Objective 3.5 Skill Sharpener

1. 843.8
2. 7,483.1
3. 728.9
4. 97.1
5. 13.4
6. 8,437.48
7. 38,378.89
8. 22.22
9. 43.43
10. 4,903.70
11. 78.939
12. 5,874.981
13. 93,939.066
14. 8,097.324
15. 8,439.524

Objective 3.6 Skill Sharpener

1. 12.9
2. 11.8
3. 166.78
4. 1,369.89
5. 579.62
6. 759.728
7. 31.9
8. 9,923.966
9. 9,489.078
10. 15.8

Objective 3.7 Skill Sharpener

1. 2.4
2. 7,990.445
3. 4,556.9
4. 9.3
5. 6,583.302
6. 132.06
7. 1,111.1
8. 791.009

9. 9.92
10. 8,666.14

Objective 3.8 Skill Sharpener

1. 76,094.6736
2. 7,512,393.081
3. 881,898.792
4. 3,812,172.719
5. 4,637,144.314
6. 79,937.68025
7. 41,579.2356
8. 151.98
9. 6,768,770.112
10. 6,794,926,884

Objective 3.9 Skill Sharpener

1. 1,420.464
2. 348.44
3. 30.7
4. 8.468962
5. 3.014876
6. 15.696
7. 10
8. 9.6625
9. 97.125
10. 30.18

Objective 3.10 Skill Sharpener

1. 6.45
2. 342.725
3. $4.\overline{33}$
4. 4,554.219667
5. 19.14
6. 96.6
7. 54.675
8. 8.08
9. 7.58
10. 433.94

Post-Test

1. 4⑤.34
2. 69⓪.00
3. 21②.932
4. 3②.893
5. 78⑤.112
6. 54⑨80

7. 6,790③532
8. 356①21
9. 100⑤6
10. 4,341⑤550
11. 34.1②30
12. 500.3②09
13. 65.9⓪10
14. ⑦50.8793
15. 3,500.5③00
16. 540.34②1
17. 442.39②8
18. 7,988.88⑨7
19. 452.52⓪3
20. 32,321.90②
21. <
22. =
23. =
24. <
25. >
26. >
27. >
28. =
29. <
30. =
31. 34.3
32. 12.4
33. 453.9
34. 45.4
35. 475.8
36. 8,347.47
37. 34.32
38. 455.45
39. 499.96
41. 3,433.334
42. 44.404
43. 434.444
44. 8.645
45. 0.333
46. 377.55
47. 486.33
48. 1,227.765
49. 54.776
50. 354,346.6984
51. 33.989
52. 3.107
53. 431.48157

54. 0.94
55. 56.013
56. 7,0229.28
57. 110.166
58. 178,425,584.8
59. 422,671,555.8
60. 369,771.9048
61. 3.726708075
62. 1.524805147
63. 1.361797753
64. 8.507175573
65. 12.41090343
66. 318.1814
67. 152.7266
68. 91.21825
69. 514.9855
70. 900.6344

CHAPTER 4 FRACTIONS

Objective 4.3 Skill Sharpener

1. $\frac{①}{2}$
2. $\frac{④}{5}$
3. $\frac{⑫}{32}$
4. $\frac{⑥}{7}$
5. $\frac{⑨}{10}$
6. $\frac{⑫}{25}$
7. $\frac{③}{4}$
8. $\frac{⑧}{12}$
9. $\frac{⑩}{12}$
10. $\frac{⑤}{9}$

Objective 4.4 Skill Sharpener

1. $\frac{3}{④}$
2. $\frac{9}{⑯}$
3. $\frac{1}{②}$
4. $\frac{5}{⑧}$
5. $\frac{17}{㉜}$
6. $\frac{4}{⑦}$
7. $\frac{3}{⑧}$
8. $\frac{9}{⑯}$
9. $\frac{22}{⑩⓪}$

10. $\frac{56}{9}$

Objective 4.5 Skill Sharpener

1. $\frac{2}{5}$ $\frac{5}{8}$ $\frac{2}{3}$
2. $\frac{1}{5}$ $\frac{2}{8}$ $\frac{6}{8}$
3. $\frac{1}{5}$ $\frac{1}{8}$ $\frac{3}{4}$
4. $\frac{1}{5}$ $\frac{1}{3}$ $\frac{2}{3}$
5. $\frac{1}{5}$ $\frac{3}{6}$ $\frac{2}{3}$
6. $\frac{1}{8}$ $\frac{1}{4}$ $\frac{3}{8}$
7. $\frac{1}{8}$ $\frac{2}{6}$ $\frac{2}{3}$
8. $\frac{3}{9}$ $\frac{2}{3}$ $\frac{4}{5}$
9. $\frac{6}{7}$ $\frac{7}{8}$ $\frac{8}{9}$
10. $\frac{1}{2}$ $\frac{3}{4}$ $\frac{5}{6}$

Objective 4.6 Skill Sharpener

1. $1\frac{2}{5}$
2. $1\frac{1}{3}$
3. $\frac{7}{8}$
4. $\frac{1}{2}$
5. $\frac{5}{9}$
6. $\frac{1}{2}$
7. $1\frac{1}{8}$
8. $\frac{4}{7}$
9. $\frac{9}{10}$
10. $\frac{24}{25}$

Objective 4.7 Skill Sharpener

1. $\frac{1}{2}$
2. $\frac{1}{3}$
3. $\frac{1}{3}$
4. $\frac{5}{12}$
5. $\frac{27}{50}$
6. $\frac{9}{16}$
7. $\frac{9}{50}$
8. $\frac{1}{16}$
9. $\frac{11}{48}$
10. $\frac{1}{4}$

Objective 4.9 Skill Sharpener

1. $3\frac{3}{5}$
2. $3\frac{7}{9}$

3. $6\frac{1}{2}$
4. $4\frac{7}{8}$
5. $3\frac{3}{10}$
6. $3\frac{3}{8}$
7. $7\frac{3}{4}$
8. $3\frac{4}{7}$
9. $3\frac{1}{10}$
10. $5\frac{1}{16}$

Objective 4.10 Skill Sharpener

1. $1\frac{1}{2}$
2. $4\frac{1}{2}$
3. $2\frac{1}{12}$
4. $1\frac{5}{8}$
5. $1\frac{3}{5}$
6. $6\frac{7}{8}$
7. $2\frac{1}{3}$
8. $2\frac{1}{11}$
9. $3\frac{3}{16}$
10. $3\frac{1}{5}$

Objective 4.11 Skill Sharpener

1. 1, 2, 4, 8
2. 1, 3, 9
3. 1, 2, 3, 4, 6, 12
4. 1, 2, 3, 6, 9, 18
5. 1, 2, 3, 4, 6, 8, 12, 24
6. 1, 2, 4, 5, 10, 20
7. 1, 2, 5, 10
8. 1, 2, 3, 6
9. 1, 2, 7, 14
10. 1, 2, 11, 22

Objective 4.12 Skill Sharpener

1. 1, 2, 4
2. 1, 2, 4
3. 1, 5
4. 1, 2, 3, 4, 6, 12
5. 1
6. 1
7. 1, 3
8. 1, 2, 4, 8
9. 1, 3
10. 1, 3

Objective 4.13 Skill Sharpener

1. 3
2. 4
3. 3
4. 3
5. 1
6. 12
7. 1
8. 1
9. 1
10. 1

Objective 4.14 Skill Sharpener

1. $\frac{3}{4}$
2. $\frac{1}{5}$
3. $\frac{1}{9}$
4. $\frac{2}{3}$
5. $\frac{1}{2}$
6. $\frac{1}{4}$
7. $\frac{1}{2}$
8. $\frac{1}{3}$
9. $\frac{1}{2}$
10. $\frac{1}{3}$

Objective 4.15 Skill Sharpener

1. P
2. P
3. I
4. I
5. P
6. P
7. I
8. I
9. P
10. P

Objective 4.16 Skill Sharpener

1. P
2. I
3. I
4. P
5. P
6. I
7. P
8. P

9. I
10. I

Objective 4.17 Skill Sharpener

1. $1\frac{1}{8}$
2. 3
3. 4
4. $1\frac{5}{7}$
5. $1\frac{1}{2}$
6. 2
7. 4
8. $3\frac{3}{4}$
9. $6\frac{1}{3}$
10. $1\frac{5}{6}$

Objective 4.18 Skill Sharpener

1. 4, 8, 12, 16, 20, 24, 28, 32, 36, 40...
2. 5, 10, 15, 20, 25, 30, 35, 40, 45, 50...
3. 6, 12, 18, 24, 30, 36, 42, 48, 54, 60..
4. 7, 14, 21, 28, 35, 42, 49, 56, 63, 70. . .
5. 8, 16, 24, 32, 40, 48, 56, 64, 72, 80. . .

Objective 4.19 Skill Sharpener

1. 4
2. 6
3. 20
4. 12
5. 14
6. 24
7. 18
8. 20
9. 36
10. 24

Objective 4.20 Skill Sharpener

1. 6
2. 4
3. 16
4. 20
5. 20

6. 16
7. 24
8. 10
9. 60
10. 8

Objective 4.21 Skill Sharpener

1. $\frac{5}{6}$
2. $1\frac{1}{6}$
3. $1\frac{5}{8}$
4. $\frac{7}{8}$
5. 1
6. $1\frac{19}{30}$
7. $\frac{5}{16}$
8. 1
9. $\frac{15}{16}$
10. $1\frac{17}{20}$

Objective 4.22 Skill Sharpener

1. $\frac{5}{12}$
2. $\frac{1}{4}$
3. $\frac{7}{15}$
4. $\frac{11}{40}$
5. $\frac{1}{2}$
6. $\frac{1}{4}$
7. $\frac{1}{6}$
8. $\frac{29}{63}$
9. $\frac{13}{72}$
10. $\frac{13}{22}$

Objective 4.23 Skill Sharpener

1. $3\frac{4}{7}$
2. 2
3. $4\frac{1}{2}$
4. $3\frac{1}{4}$
5. 2
6. $1\frac{7}{8}$
7. $2\frac{5}{8}$
8. $5\frac{23}{24}$
9. $\frac{39}{40}$
10. $\frac{28}{33}$

Objective 4.24 Skill Sharpener

1. $\frac{29}{9}$
2. $\frac{69}{8}$
3. $\frac{11}{4}$
4. $\frac{44}{6}$
5. $\frac{14}{11}$
6. $\frac{484}{50}$
7. $\frac{81}{12}$
8. $\frac{50}{9}$
9. $\frac{126}{10}$
10. $\frac{7}{2}$

Objective 4.25 Skill Sharpener

1. $\frac{1}{2}$
2. $\frac{1}{12}$
3. $\frac{7}{10}$
4. $\frac{5}{18}$
5. $\frac{1}{4}$
6. $\frac{1}{10}$
7. $\frac{3}{16}$
8. $\frac{5}{24}$
9. $\frac{7}{90}$
10. $\frac{6}{35}$

Objective 4.26 Skill Sharpener

1. $\frac{1}{9}$
2. $\frac{1}{9}$
3. $\frac{1}{4}$
4. $\frac{1}{8}$
5. $\frac{10}{21}$
6. $\frac{1}{8}$
7. $\frac{7}{12}$
8. $\frac{5}{8}$
9. $\frac{1}{15}$
10. $\frac{1}{2}$

Objective 4.27 Skill Sharpener

1. 8
2. $\frac{3}{5}$
3. $3\frac{1}{5}$
4. $1\frac{2}{3}$

5. 5

6. $1\frac{2}{3}$

7. 6

8. $1\frac{2}{3}$

9. $2\frac{13}{16}$

10. $\frac{5}{9}$

Objective 4.28 Skill Sharpener

1. $2\frac{1}{3}$

2. $1\frac{13}{20}$

3. $\frac{7}{10}$

4. $\frac{111}{128}$

5. 2

6. $2\frac{13}{16}$

7. $\frac{38}{77}$

8. $7\frac{21}{64}$

9. $2\frac{6}{7}$

10. 5

Objective 4.29 Skill Sharpener

1. $1\frac{1}{2}$

2. $1\frac{5}{16}$

3. $1\frac{5}{27}$

4. $2\frac{1}{4}$

5. 2

6. $2\frac{1}{16}$

7. $6\frac{4}{5}$

8. $2\frac{2}{5}$

9. $4\frac{67}{160}$

10. $3\frac{11}{15}$

Post-Test

1. $\frac{①}{2}$

2. $\frac{㉓}{48}$

3. $\frac{②}{10}$

4. $\frac{⑥}{12}$

5. $\frac{①②⑤}{1000}$

6. $\frac{12}{⑭}$

7. $\frac{5}{㊽}$

8. $\frac{15}{⑯}$

9. $\frac{7}{⑧}$

10. $\frac{3}{④}$

11. $\frac{1}{6}$ $\frac{1}{5}$ $\frac{1}{4}$ $\frac{1}{3}$ $\frac{1}{2}$

12. $\frac{3}{8}$ $\frac{7}{16}$ $\frac{1}{2}$ $\frac{9}{16}$ $\frac{3}{4}$

13. $\frac{11}{16}$ $\frac{12}{16}$ $\frac{12}{15}$ $\frac{7}{8}$ $\frac{9}{10}$

14. $\frac{6}{15}$ $\frac{4}{9}$ $\frac{3}{4}$ $\frac{4}{5}$ $\frac{10}{12}$

15. $\frac{1}{2}$ $\frac{2}{3}$ $\frac{3}{4}$ $\frac{4}{5}$ $\frac{5}{6}$

16. 1

17. 1

18. $1\frac{1}{16}$

19. $\frac{5}{12}$

20. $\frac{9}{32}$

21. $\frac{1}{50}$

22. $\frac{1}{4}$

23. $\frac{3}{10}$

24. $\frac{1}{2}$

25. $\frac{2}{5}$

26. 4

27. $4\frac{1}{8}$

28. 28

29. 19

30. $5\frac{1}{2}$

31. $10\frac{1}{2}$

32. $53\frac{1}{2}$

33. $\frac{3}{16}$

34. $36\frac{5}{8}$

35. $10\frac{4}{5}$

36. 1, 2, 3, 4, 6, 12

37. 1, 2, 4, 8, 16

38. 1, 2, 3, 6

39. 1, 2, 5, 10

40. 1, 2, 4, 8

41. 6

42. 6

43. 3

44. 8

45. 4

46. $\frac{1}{2}$

47. $\frac{1}{3}$

48. $\frac{1}{16}$

49. $\frac{1}{3}$

50. $\frac{7}{8}$

51. $\frac{2}{1}$ or 2

52. $\frac{4}{1}$ or 4

53. $1\frac{2}{5}$

54. $\frac{4}{1}$ or 4

55. $\frac{9}{1}$ or 9

56. 12

57. 9

58. 14

59. 20

60. 10

61. 12

62. 48

63. 24

64. 48

65. 20

66. $\frac{11}{12}$

67. $1\frac{1}{2}$

68. $1\frac{5}{14}$

69. $1\frac{2}{15}$

70. $\frac{13}{16}$

71. $\frac{13}{24}$

72. $\frac{11}{24}$

73. $\frac{1}{6}$

74. $\frac{7}{12}$

75. $\frac{3}{16}$

76. $1\frac{3}{4}$

77. $3\frac{2}{3}$

78. $\frac{7}{8}$

79. $3\frac{2}{5}$

80. $1\frac{7}{8}$

81. $\frac{9}{8}$

82. $\frac{33}{9}$

83. $\frac{7}{2}$

84. $\frac{51}{4}$

85. $\frac{21}{8}$

86. $\frac{1}{2}$

87. $\frac{5}{12}$

88. $\frac{3}{10}$

89. $\frac{5}{12}$

90. $\frac{21}{32}$

91. $\frac{7}{20}$

92. $\frac{2}{9}$

93. $\frac{2}{9}$

94. $\frac{7}{10}$

95. $\frac{3}{4}$

96. $1\frac{1}{8}$

97. $1\frac{1}{2}$

98. $1\frac{19}{21}$

99. $1\frac{7}{8}$

100. $1\frac{5}{16}$

CHAPTER 5 RATIOS AND PROPORTIONS

Objective 5.3 Skill Sharpener

1. equal
2. not equal
3. equal
4. equal
5. equal
6. not equal
7. not equal
8. equal
9. not equal
10. equal

Objective 5.4 Skill Sharpener

1. x = 24
2. x = 200
3. x = 578
4. x = 4
5. x = 30,000
6. x = 8
7. $x = 7.\overline{33}$
8. x = 4.5
9. x = 129.85074
10. x = 0.78

Objective 5.5 Skill Sharpener

1. 3 mL
2. 4
3. 2
4. $0.2\overline{66}$
5. 1 mL
6. 61.25%
7. $35 per hour
8. 11.43%
9. 3.9473684%
10. 18.63%

Post-Test

1. 7:8
2. 3:12
3. 33:66
4. 9:27
5. 20:30
6. equal
7. not equal
8. not equal
9. not equal
10. equal
11. x = 3
12. x = 360
13. x = 18
14. x = 270,000
15. x = 2
16. 7.5 mL
17. 3.36%
18. 10 mL
19. 6 mL
20. 20%
21. 83.87%
22. $1\frac{1}{2}$ mL
23. 11.88%
24. yes
25. 0.156 second

CHAPTER 6 PERCENTS

Objective 6.2 Skill Sharpener

1. 37.5%
2. 9.32%
3. 183.2%
4. 90.83%
5. 233.23%
6. 33.34%
7. 4,543.243%
8. 123.2%
9. 98.23%
10. 66.76%

Objective 6.3 Skill Sharpener

1. 0.34
2. 3.45
3. 0.039
4. 0.12232
5. 0.75532
6. 0.99032
7. 0.312594
8. 0.54433
9. 0.0845
10. 0.92322

Objective 6.4 Skill Sharpener

1. 262.5
2. 5.18
3. 247.5
4. 3.84
5. 800
6. 2.85
7. 7.5
8. 29.92
9. 42.25
10. 14.8%
11. 33%
12. 20%
13. 6.$\overline{66}$%
14. 83.$\overline{33}$%
15. 25%
16. 30%
17. 18.42105%
18. 3.40909%
19. 64%
20. 35.71428%

Objective 6.5 Skill Sharpener

1. 110.5
2. 112.5
3. 40.625
4. 26.2808
5. 14.592
6. 513.086
7. 1.35
8. 6.93
9. 63.365
10. 20.068
11. 12.5%
12. 74%
13. 22%
14. 11%
15. 52%
16. 36%
17. 7%

18. 45%
19. 97%
20. 2.56%

Post-Test

1. 45%
2. 78%
3. 89%
4. 91%
5. 33.41%
6. 25.56%
7. 87.3%
8. 11.2%
9. 49.4%
10. 100%
11. 0.34
12. 0.57
13. 0.12
14. 0.9
15. 0.43
16. 0.7567
17. 0.3944
18. 0.11901
19. 0.85554
20. 0.2245
21. 262.5
22. 20.145
23. 1188
24. 29.975
25. 10,511.847
26. 0.06
27. 3.366
28. 11,661
29. 21.44
30. 2.7
31. 45%
32. 25%
33. 13%
34. 72.996479%
35. 14%
36. 32%
37. 3%
38. 12%
39. 1.8%
40. 9%
41. $652.91
42. $1,185.75
43. 104
44. $17.70
45. $30
46. 65%
47. 53.14%
48. $134.06
49. 31 cents
50. 37%

CHAPTER 7 CONVERSIONS

Objective 7.1 Skill Sharpener

1. $\frac{19}{50}$
2. $\frac{97}{100}$
3. $\frac{233}{1000}$
4. $\frac{1}{8}$
5. $\frac{1}{4}$
6. $\frac{3}{4}$
7. $\frac{9}{10}$
8. $1\frac{23}{100}$
9. $2\frac{3}{4}$
10. $3\frac{1}{2}$

Objective 7.2 Skill Sharpener

1. 34%
2. 25%
3. 87%
4. 67%
5. 39%
6. 20%
7. 90%
8. 12.3%
9. 123%
10. 278%

Objective 7.3 Skill Sharpener

1. 0.5
2. 0.66
3. 0.8
4. 0.4375
5. 0.9
6. 0.32
7. 0.375
8. 0.5
9. $0.\overline{33}$
10. 0.125

Objective 7.4 Skill Sharpener

1. 80%
2. 66.$\overline{66}$%
3. 12.5%
4. 85.7%
5. 33.$\overline{33}$%
6. 33.$\overline{33}$%
7. 51.$\overline{11}$%
8. 30%
9. 43.75%
10. 25%

Objective 7.5 Skill Sharpener

1. $\frac{23}{100}$
2. $\frac{9}{20}$
3. $\frac{9}{10}$
4. $\frac{1}{2}$
5. $\frac{33}{100}$
6. $\frac{13}{20}$
7. $\frac{3}{5}$
8. $\frac{3}{25}$
9. $\frac{9}{100}$
10. $1\frac{1}{4}$

Objective 7.6 Skill Sharpener

1. 0.32
2. 0.15
3. 0.67
4. 3.24
5. 0.03
6. 0.13
7. 0.91
8. 0.0038
9. 0.009
10. 0.12

Objective 7.7 Skill Sharpener

1. 0.056
2. 0.26
3. 0.034
4. 24,000
5. 230
6. 500
7. 0.029
8. 3.4

9. 2,300
10. 125

Objective 7.8 Skill Sharpener

1. 1.07
2. 112.5
3. 1
4. 1
5. 240
6. 1
7. 8
8. 8
9. 32
10. 60

Objective 7.9 Skill Sharpener

1. 1
2. $1\frac{1}{3}$
3. 8
4. 8
5. 2
6. 3
7. 2
8. 360
9. $1\frac{1}{2}$
10. 9

Objective 7.10 Skill Sharpener

1. 360
2. 500
3. 720
4. 180
5. 15
6. 60
7. 2
8. 60
9. 2
10. 2

Post-Test

1. $\frac{11}{25}$
2. $\frac{17}{25}$
3. $\frac{23}{100}$
4. $\frac{11}{100}$
5. $\frac{49}{50}$

6. 46%
7. 12.5%
8. 33%
9. 87%
10. 58%
11. 0.44
12. 0.9
13. 0.68
14. 0.55
15. 0.8
16. 74.5%
17. 37.5%
18. $6.\overline{66}$%
19. $66.\overline{66}$%
20. $36.\overline{36}$
21. $\frac{17}{50}$
22. $\frac{57}{100}$
23. $\frac{87}{100}$
24. $\frac{33}{50}$
25. $\frac{3}{25}$
26. 0.13
27. 0.61
28. 0.59
29. 0.31
30. 0.98
31. 3000
32. 1200
33. 1.3
34. 595
35. 240
36. 2
37. 2
38. 3
39. 16
40. 12

CHAPTER 8 MEDICAL DOSAGE CALCULATIONS

Objective 8.1 Skill Sharpener

1. Trade name: Comvax
   Generic name: Haemophilus b Conjugate and Hepatitis B Vaccine
   Manufacturer: Merck and Company
   NDC number: 0006-4898-00
   Dosage strength: 7.5 mcg of Hib, 125 mcg Neisseria meningitides, and 5 mcg of hepatitis B surface antigen
   Drug form: liquid
   Usual adult dose: 0.5 mL
   Amount enclosed: 10 vials
   Prescription warning: not seen
   Expiration date: not seen
   Lot number: not seen

2. Trade name: MMR II
   Generic name: MMR Virus Vaccine Live
   Manufacturer: Merck
   NDC number: 0006-4749-00
   Dosage strength: 25 mcg
   Drug form: liquid for injection
   Usual adult dose: 0.5 mL
   Amount enclosed: 1 dose vial
   Prescription warning: Federal (USA) law prohibits dispensing without prescription.
   Expiration date: not seen
   Lot number: not seen

3. Trade name: Mevacor
   Generic name: Lovastatin
   Manufacturer: Merck
   NDC number: 0006-0731-61
   Dosage strength: 20 mg
   Drug form: tablets
   Usual adult dose: not seen
   Amount enclosed: 60 tablets
   Prescription warning: not seen
   Expiration date: December 1997
   Lot number: B3143

4. Trade name: Singulair
   Generic name: Montelukast Sodium
   Manufacturer: Merck
   NDC number: 0006-0711-30
   Dosage strength: 4 mg
   Drug form: tablets
   Usual adult dose: This is a pediatric medication with child dose noted.
   Amount enclosed: 30 tablets
   Prescription warning: not seen

Expiration date: not seen
Lot number: not seen

5. Trade name: Celebrex
   Generic name: celecoxib
   Manufacturer: Pfizer, Searle
   NDC number: 0025-1520-31
   (100 mg) 0025-1525-31 (200 mg)
   Dosage strength: 100 mg or
   200 mg
   Drug form: tablet
   Usual adult dose: not seen
   Amount enclosed: 100 tablets
   Prescription warning: not seen
   Expiration date: not seen
   Lot number: not seen

Objective 8.2 Skill Sharpener

1. Diptheria and tetanus toxoids
   and acellular pertussis vaccine
   adsorbed
2. Infanrix
3. No. It is on the back of the
   package.
4. 0.5 mL
5. not seen
6. 5 mL
7. not seen
8. 58160-840-11
9. drug form, usual dose, expiration
   date, lot number
10. This is a pediatric medication
    (vaccine).

Objective 8.3 Skill Sharpener

1. Lane Kennamer
2. 205-555-1212
3. Dora Reid
4. Tussionex Suspension
5. not shown
6. 240 mL
7. Yes, two.
8. yes
9. take thou
10. Take one teaspoon by mouth
    every 12 hours.

Objective 8.4 Skill Sharpener

1. 3 mL
2. 2 mL
3. 8 mL
4. 6 mL
5. 9 mL

Objective 8.5 Skill Sharpener

1. remaining: 300 mL
   infused: 700 mL
2. remaining: 500 mL
   infused: 500 mL
3. remaining: 200 mL
   infused: 800 mL
4. remaining: 500 mL
   infused: 0
5. remaining: 100 mL
   infused: 900 mL

Objective 8.6 Skill Sharpener

1. 10 gtts/min
2. 22 gtts/min
3. 23 gtts/min
4. 62 gtts/min
5. 50 gtts/min

Objective 8.7 Skill Sharpener

Concentration of solutions

1.	4	4%
2.	12.5	12.5%
3.	50	50%
4.	10	10%
5.	9	9%

Percent strength

1. 0.6 gm
2. 6.75 gm
3. 5.25 gm
4. 15 gm
5. 1.08 gm

Objective 8.8 Skill Sharpener

1. 6 mL
2. 1.3 mL
3. 3.25 mL

4. $1\frac{1}{2}$ mL
5. 3
6. $0.2\overline{66}$ mL
7. 0.5 mL
8. 10 mL
9. 0.8 mL
10. 1 mL

Objective 8.9 Skill Sharpener

1. Take one tablespoon of the cough syrup by mouth.
2. Take 1 teaspoon of an elixir by mouth four times a day.
3. Take 1 tablet every 4 hours as needed for nausea.
4. Take 2 capsules by mouth each day until gone (7 days).
5. Allow one tablet to dissolve under your tongue as needed for chest pain.
6. Take 3 tablets by mouth three times a day.
7. Take 2 tablets by mouth twice a day.
8. Drink 1 glass before bedtime then take nothing by mouth until after the test.
9. Take 2 tablespoons of the medication after meals.
10. Take 2 teaspoons by mouth every other day.

Post-Test

1. NDC number
2. Manufacturer
3. Warning
4. Trade name
5. Generic name
6. Usual adult dose
7. Dosage strength
8. Drug form
9. Total amount enclosed
10. Lot number
11. Physician's name
12. Patient's name
13. Refill blank
14. Designation to label
15. Generic substitution allowed
16. Dispense as written
17. Instructions for taking medication
18. Subscription
19. Physician address
20. Patient address
21. $1\frac{1}{2}$ mL
22. 5 mL
23. 2 mL
24. 1 mL
25. 4 mL
26. 1 mL
27. 4 mL
28. 2 mL
29. $\frac{1}{2}$ mL
30. $2\frac{1}{2}$ mL
31. 50 mL
32. 600 mL
33. 200 mL
34. 200 mL
35. 500 mL
36. 300 mL
37. 400 mL
38. 800 mL
39. 700 mL
40. 100 mL
41. 21 gtts/min
42. 250 gtts/min
43. 10 gtts/min
44. 50 gtts/min
45. 33 gtts/min
46. 8   8%
47. 12   12%
48. 25   25%
49. 15   15%
50. 3   3%
51. 0.36 gm
52. 4 gm
53. 2.7 gm
54. 0.2 gm
55. 0.05 gm
56. 3.75 mL
57. 3 mL
58. 7 mL
59. 10 mL
60. 0.6 mL

61. Place one tablet under your tongue as needed for chest pain.
62. Take 3 tablets by mouth three times/day.
63. Take 3 tablets twice a day until gone (7 days).
64. Take 1 teaspoon twice a day.
65. Take 2 teaspoons by mouth twice a day.

CHAPTER 9 WEIGHTS AND MEASURES

Objective 9.1 Skill Sharpener

1. 135 lb
2. 75 lb
3. 148 lb
4. 248 lb
5. 35 lb

Objective 9.2 Skill Sharpener

1. 100 kg
2. 80 kg
3. 18 kg
4. 5 kg
5. 89 kg
6. 70 kg
7. 41 kg
8. 55 kg
9. 91 kg
10. 3 kg
11. 121 lb
12. 220 lb
13. 242 lb
14. 48 lb
15. 26 lb
16. 198 lb
17. 341 lb
18. 176 lb
19. 275 lb
20. 286 lb

Objective 9.3 Skill Sharpener

1. $2\frac{1}{2}''$
2. $4\frac{3}{8}''$
3. $3\frac{3}{4}''$
4. $1\frac{15}{16}''$
5. $2''$
6. $2\frac{3}{8}''$
7. $1\frac{3}{8}''$
8. $4''$
9. $5\frac{1}{4}''$
10. $4\frac{1}{16}''$

Objective 9.4 Skill Sharpener

1. 3 cm or 30 mm
2. 82 mm or 8.2 cm
3. 79 mm or 7.9 cm
4. 120 mm or 12 cm
5. 40 mm or 4 cm
6. $2\frac{1}{2}$ cm or 25 mm
7. $11\frac{1}{2}$ cm or 115 mm
8. 65 mm or 6.5 cm
9. 19 mm or 1.9 cm
10. $3\frac{1}{2}$ cm or 35 mm

Objective 9.5 Skill Sharpener

1. 3.05 m
2. 0.84 m
3. 2.82 m
4. 1.37 m
5. 19.82 m
6. 62.32 ft
7. 8.2 ft
8. 42.64 ft
9. 367.36 ft
10. 275.52 ft
11. 36″
12. 24″
13. 30″
14. 63″
15. 59.06″

Objective 9.6 Skill Sharpener

1. 99.0°F
2. 99.8°F
3. 99.2°F
4. 101.2°F
5. 98.4°F
6. 102.4°F
7. 98.6°F
8. 96.8°F

9. 99.4°F
10. 100°F

Objective 9.7 Skill Sharpener

1. 48.9°C
2. 5°C
3. 37.6°C
4. 38.5°C
5. 39.4°C
6. 89.6°F
7. 188.6°F
8. 55.2°F
9. 109.4°F
10. 131°F

Objective 9.8 Skill Sharpener

1. 0.9 m²
2. 1.1 m²
3. 1.34 m²
4. 0.60 m²
5. 1.2 m²
6. 1.95 m²
7. 1.75 m²
8. 0.6 m²
9. 0.27 m²
10. 0.5 m²

Post-Test

1. 195 lb
2. 115 lb
3. 80 lb
4. 48 lb
5. 160 lb
6. 68 kg
7. 101 kg
8. 11 kg
9. 18 kg
10. 75 kg
11. 150 lb
12. 20 lb
13. 713 lb
14. 165 lb
15. 200 lb
16. $5\frac{1}{4}''$
17. $2\frac{5}{8}''$
18. $1\frac{3}{8}''$

19. 4″
20. $3\frac{1}{8}''$
21. 5.18 meters
22. 8.26 meters
23. 182.88 cm
24. 10.16 cm
25. 63.5 mm
26. 9.84 ft
27. 39.36 ft
28. 108.24 ft
29. 17.7 in
30. 23 in
31. 104°F
32. 95.6°F
33. 101.2°F
34. 100.8°F
35. 98.6°F
36. 37°C
37. 25.6°C
38. 38.9°C
39. 12.8°C
40. 676.7°C
41. 53.6°F
42. 93.2°F
43. 131°F
44. 71.6°F
45. 244.4°F
46. 0.68 m²
47. 0.22 m²
48. 0.98 m²
49. 2 m²
50. 0.18 m²

CHAPTER 10 MEASURING INTAKE AND OUTPUT

Objective 10.2 Skill Sharpener

1. 100 mL
2. 140 mL
3. 210 mL
4. 180 mL
5. 230 mL
6. 130 mL
7. 150 mL
8. 220 mL
9. 310 mL
10. 160 mL

Objective 10.3 Skill Sharpener

1. 1,800 mL
2. 1,700 mL
3. 2,120 mL
4. 2,400 mL
5. 1,750 mL
6. 2,450 mL
7. 2,145 mL
8. 2,100 mL
9. 1,700 mL
10. 2,300 mL

Objective 10.4 Skill Sharpener

1. 360 mL
2. 250 mL
3. 860 mL
4. 3,030 mL
5. 1,680 mL

Objective 10.5 Skill Sharpener

1. 50 mL retention
2. 440 mL retention
3. balance
4. 3,510 mL
5. 2,610 mL

Post-Test

1. 200 mL
2. 150 mL
3. 350 mL
4. 625 mL
5. 400 mL
6. 2,100 mL
7. 2,550 mL
8. 1,800 mL
9. 1,650 mL
10. 2,400 mL
11. 960 mL
12. 740 mL
13. 960 mL
14. 500 mL

15. 850 mL
16. 240 mL
17. 480 mL
18. 65 mL
19. 160 mL
20. 90 mL
21. retained 100 mL
22. retained 20 mL
23. 50 mL more output than intake
24. 145 mL more output than intake
25. retained 50 mL

APPENDIX E FINAL SUMMATIVE EVALUATION

1. 144 lb
2. $65\frac{1}{2}''$
3. A
4. one
5. every 6 hours
6. Ceclor
7. Lilly
8. Lasix
9. 8 mL
10. once
11. 60
12. 30 days
13. 68°F–77°F
14. 2920 mL
15. 2920 mL
16. b
17. 25 gtts/min
18. 3 hours and 20 minutes
19. 20%
20. one each of 2 mg and 1 mg tablets
21. 3 times a day—breakfast, lunch, dinner
22. 2 tablets
23. 9 tablets
24. 0.8 mL
25. 9 mL

INDEX

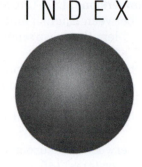